M.Shepherd

Paul ____

Case Presentati

Titles in the series

Case Presentations in Accident and Emergency Medicine
Case Presentations in Anaesthesia and Intensive Care
Case Presentations in Arterial Disease
Case Presentations in Clinical Geriatric Medicine
Case Presentations in Endocrinology and Diabetes
Case Presentations in Gastrointestinal Disease
Case Presentations in General Surgery
Case Presentations in Heart Disease (Second Edition)
Case Presentations in Medical Ophthalmology
Case Presentations in Neurology
Case Presentations in Obstetrics and Gynaecology
Case Presentations in Otolaryngology
Case Presentations in Paediatrics
Case Presentations in Psychiatry
Case Presentations in Respiratory Medicine

Titles in preparation

Case Presentations in Urology

Case Presentations in Psychiatry

Dinesh Bhugra, MSc MBBS, MRCPsych, MPhil
MRC Social and Community Psychiatry Unit, Institute of Psychiatry,
London

Stephen Potts, MA, BMBCh, MRCPsych
University Department of Psychiatry, Royal Edinburgh Hospital,
Edinburgh

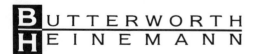

Butterworth-Heinemann Ltd
Linacre House, Jordan Hill, Oxford OX2 8DP

 PART OF REED INTERNATIONAL BOOKS

OXFORD   LONDON   BOSTON
MUNICH   NEW DELHI   SINGAPORE   SYDNEY
TOKYO   TORONTO   WELLINGTON

First published 1993

British Library Cataloguing in Publication Data
A catalogue record for this book is available from the British Library

ISBN 0 7506 1542 7

Library of Congress Cataloguing in Publication Data
A catalogue record for this book is available from the Library of Congress

Typeset and Illustrated by TecSet Ltd, Wallington, Surrey
Printed and bound in Great Britain by Biddles Ltd, Guildford and
Kings Lynn

Preface

To be a good psychiatrist one needs clinical skills, empathy and knowledge. Membership of the Royal College of Psychiatrists is only one step in the growth towards becoming a good clinician. While it may be true to some extent that good clinicians are born but not created, it is important to remember that clinical skills can certainly be polished. This book will not turn its readers into psychiatrists overnight, but will enable them to hone their learning and practice dealing with day-to-day clinical situations as well as prepare them for the membership examinations.

Now that both parts of the membership examinations have clinical components, the candidate has to apply different skills to various parts of the examination. Whereas in the first part the candidate has to demonstrate his/her grasp of psychopathology, the second part deals with management issues, whether in clinical cases or in the patient management problems (PMPs or case vignettes).

This book is divided into four sections. The first section has two chapters devoted to polishing up clinical skills and getting ready for the examination itself. The second section forms the major part of the book with 60 PMPs—with questions and answers including decision trees and references. This section has 15 sets of 'papers' with four vignettes each. It is worth bearing in mind that some examiners prefer to focus on PMPs which are unlikely to be seen in the clinical examination itself, e.g. child psychiatry or mental handicap. The third section has five cases illustrating the problems and solutions for MRCPsych I—

which focuses largely on psychopathology. The last section has five cases in the longer format of MRCPsych II, and deals more with issues of management and prognosis. It will be a useful preparatory exercise if candidates can get together in a group or in twos and threes to discuss PMPs.

We would like to thank Dr Clive Meux for his kindness and help in formulating forensic PMPs and their responses, and to various trainees who helped with corrections.

We should like to acknowledge our appreciation for Mr Paul Valentine at Coombe's Medical Library at St. Bernard's Hospital, Southall, and Ms Sue Floate, Librarian at the Royal College of Psychiatrists. We are greatly indebted to Mrs Maureen Trott for her secretarial skills and patience.

Dinesh Bhugra
Stephen Potts

Contents

1 General approach to clinical examination

Introduction

Until recently, Part I of the MRCPsych examination had no clinical content. In 1987 a clinical examination, focusing on issues of assessment and diagnosis, was added, and corresponding adjustments were made to the clinical element of Part II. For the Part I clinical examination the Royal College of Psychiatrists' *Regulations for the MRCPsych examinations* (p. 8) state:

> The clinical examination will test basic skills of psychiatric assessment: the ability to relate to the patient, to take a history and examine the mental state, and to exercise judgment in bringing the relevant information together to make a succinct and accurate assessment. A detailed plan of management is not required. Candidates will be expected to examine a case or cases which may be drawn from any aspect of adult general psychiatry for fifty minutes. During the thirty minute interview with a pair of Examiners, candidates are expected to further interview the patient for about ten minutes in the presence of Examiners. The main areas of assessment are the candidate's ability to establish a satisfactory relationship with the patient, take a full psychiatric history, carry out an accurate mental state examination, make appropriate deductions from the information available to him, and come to a conclusion about the differential diagnosis of the disorder from which the patient is suffering.

Part II has two clinical elements, the clinical examination and the oral or viva voce. The clinical examination lasts for a total of

90 minutes, of which an hour is allocated for the patient interview, and the candidate is then examined for 30 minutes by two examiners. It is the most important part of the examination since failure in this part means automatic failure of the whole examination. After hearing the candidate's presentation of the case the examiners will discuss with the candidate his or her assessment, management plan, and view of the prognosis. They will also ask the candidate to re-interview the patient in their presence, to elicit specific psychopathology. The discussion with the examiners will cover assessment (overall view, findings on examination, diagnosis and differential diagnosis, and the supposed aetiological factors); management (further enquiries, investigations, and treatment, both short-term and long-term) and prognosis.

The oral examination now lasts for 30 minutes, and is conducted by a second pair of examiners, who will present the candidate with patient management problems (PMPs, also known as vignettes), which they usually prepare in advance. The College guidelines state that 'Questions may be asked on any aspect of psychiatric disorders *and their management.*' (Royal College of Psychiatrists' *Regulations for the MRCPsych Examination* p. 22).

In any clinical encounter, the examiners assess not only the interview skills of the candidate but also his or her more general clinical qualities. In considering the former they are likely to assess the candidate's technique in approaching clinical problems with a systematic, comprehensive and flexible approach. The candidate should therefore emphasize his or her control of the patient's interview without turning it into an interrogation. Hence, for example, open ended questions followed by summary statements to the patient are a good clinical technique. While assessing the general clinical qualities of the candidate, the focus is on whether the candidate is safe, sensitive, empathic, objective, and able to work effectively while anxious; and whether the candidate acknowledges other professionals' skills. This book will not provide readers with all these qualities, but will help to train candidates to ask and answer questions in a systematic manner.

This book is primarily intended to help candidates prepare for the oral examination, and presents 60 PMPs within 15 sets of

4, with appropriate answers and decision trees. It can also be used to prepare for the clinical examinations, of both the Part I and Part II examinations, especially the management aspects of the clinical examination in Part II. To this end five longer case histories are set out, with questions and answers, for each level of the examination.

Preparation for the clinical examination

Candidates should bring their knowledge up to date, since in face-to-face encounters the examiners are most likely to ask about the latest scientific papers. Having revised adequately candidates should spend some time in the library reviewing back-issues of the *British Journal of Psychiatry*, *Psychological Medicine*, the *American Journal of Psychiatry*, and *Archives of General Psychiatry*, as well as the *British Medical Journal* and the *Lancet*. They should certainly be familiar with the recent relevant editorials and review articles in these journals. Review articles also appear in the *British Journal of Hospital Medicine* and various collected volumes of such articles (e.g. *Comprehensive Psychiatry*, *Contemporary Psychiatry*). Exercises with short answer questions (SAQs) will enable candidates to present their discussions in a concise manner (see Bhugra, 1990).

Candidates should try to practise presenting cases under examination conditions mimicking both the clinical and oral examinations, to their consultants, clinical tutors and senior registrars. The cases should be presented to as many different people as possible because that will expose candidates to different lines of questioning. It is better to be harassed in the rehearsals than on the day. Candidates can prepare by thinking of the questions that are likely to be asked. They should try to work on any possible negative feedback. Sometimes recording the interview and performance can make candidates' handicaps glaringly obvious and therefore easy to correct. The presentation should be practised in a format with which candidates feel familiar and comfortable. In their psychiatric training candidates will have developed their own style; they should adhere to it, making sure that it adequately covers all areas of assessment. The decision tree model employed in this book (see Chapter 2) gives an idea of the problems that may be asked about and how to deal with these. The Institute of Psychiatry guidelines (1975) on eliciting and recording clinical information are excellent for preparing the assessment.

The examination is often said to be an interview for joining a club. Candidates should, therefore, dress smartly and comfortably. Examiners are, in general, interested in middle-of-the-road sensible psychiatry; hence candidates should not be too esoteric in manner, dress or the content of what they say. Men should dress in comfortable lounge suits with a light shirt and a sombre tie. College or club ties should be avoided (the examiner may belong to the rival institution). Women should avoid flamboyant outfits, which may give the wrong impression. Candidates should try to contain their anxiety and appear relaxed, even if they do not feel it: as noted earlier, examiners are looking for someone who is able to contain his or her anxieties. Appropriate dress thus avoids an unnecessary additional source of anxiety, adding to a feeling of relaxation which will enable candidates to demonstrate their competence as good psychiatrists.

Clinical Examination

Having arrived at the examination centre in good time, candidates should avoid getting into discussion with agitated or super-confident show-offs among fellow candidates in the waiting room. They should make a note of the examiners' names, which are usually on display in the waiting room. When asked to interview the patient before the examiners, candidates will get off to a bad start if they try to introduce the examiners to the patient but cannot recall their names. When introduced to the patient by the invigilators, candidates should make it quite clear to the patient that it is they who are on trial and not the patient, and as a reflection of the time limit, some of the questions may seem direct and abrupt. They should always remain polite to the patient. Even when the patient is a difficult case, it is almost always possible to gain some information. Candidates should let the invigilator know if they are unable to gather any information at all. They should set some time aside to interview the informant if this has been arranged. After the initial formalities most of the time will be spent on history taking and Mental State Examination. Candidates will need to practice sufficiently to know how best to divide their time and to learn how quickly it passes. Wherever indicated they should try to do a physical examination even if it is brief and selective. After obtaining the information required they should leave some time to organize their thoughts and ask any supplementary questions of the patient. Holden (1987) offers some sensible practical advice on examination techniques in psychiatry.

When with the examiners, candidates should not rush in, talk too quickly or too loudly—all of which are suggestive of anxiety. They should try to relax and smile appropriately. Since no written information is asked for by the examiners, any notes are for the candidate's guidance alone and they should be referred to as an *aide-mémoire*—not read out. The examiners will ask candidates to present their assessment, following which they may ask them to demonstrate certain signs or symptoms. The candidate should have prepared the patient for such an eventuality and introduced the patient to the examiners, explaining what he or she is going to do. The examiners are interested in observing the candidate's rapport with the patient and his or her clinical style. Once the interview is over the candidate should thank the patient and escort him or her out. The rest of the discussion is likely to focus on management and prognosis. This is where most of the confusion occurs in the examination. The examiners may wish to know the prognosis of that particular patient, whereas the candidate may be focusing on general prognostic factors for the condition the patient suffers from, or vice versa. Thus, it is of paramount importance that the candidate is absolutely clear as to what is expected. If it is not clear he or she should ask the examiners to clarify. Candidates should not be bullied by the examiners or bully them. They should try to adhere to their assessment unless given some additional information or unless they realize that they have missed some vital point. It is perfectly acceptable to be flexible, but not obsequiously so. At the end of the clinical examination, the candidate should thank the examiners before leaving.

Patient management problems (PMPs)

Candidates should try to confine themselves to the decision trees with which they have become familiar through practice and preparation. If the examiner gives a thumb-nail sketch and asks for the candidate's assessment, it is easy to get into the 'assessment mode' if it has been practised well, and to present the answers accordingly.

Waiting

The principles discussed earlier apply here as well. While waiting, candidates should talk to each other about the PMPs being asked, unless they find this makes them even more anxious. This will enable them to judge the examiners' techniques and favourite questions. 'Bully' candidates should not be allowed to undermine confidence and spread rumours while discussing difficult questions. Their ambition appears to be to frighten everyone around them.

Subjects

On average the examiners will try to cover at least four PMPs during the half hour. The emphasis is often on topics and clinical conditions that are less likely to be seen in clinical examinations. Some examiners will, therefore, prefer PMPs from mental handicap, child psychiatry, liaison psychiatry, emergency psychiatry and forensic psychiatry. Others may prefer cases from their own clinical experience. The examiners have instructions to steer away from areas of their own personal interest, so although candidates may recall the examiners' specialist fields when they see their names, it is not crucial to know this.

Style

The contents of PMPs and the subsequent questions will vary in style with different examiners. Some examiners like to give a detailed case vignette and then ask a limited number of questions. Others may, however, follow a thumb-nail sketch with increasingly difficult questions, adding information and taking the candidate down one decision path. Others may use a combination of the two techniques. The answer should be structured, informative and as interesting as the candidate can make it. The emphasis should be on practical decisions, but applying appropriate theoretical knowledge and justifying the decisions. Very occasionally candidates may be asked a question which completely throws them e.g. 'You have two years to close your hospital. How would you proceed'? They should take heart. This usually means that they have already done enough to pass, so the best response is for them to relax and try to think on their feet as they might in a less formal setting.

Keywords

For PMPs, the examiners often give a clue in the age, gender, race or occupation of the patient. It is vital that candidates keep these in mind while structuring their answers. If the examiners are talking about a 14-year-old patient with anorexia nervosa candidates would lose marks if their answers focused on adult anorexic patients. Keywords are discussed further in the next chapter.

Technique

A good technique in oral examinations is for candidates to be able to lead the examiner in asking the questions to which they know the answers without being too obvious about it.

The examiners may have had a long day and be feeling tired and bored, so a little banter may help in formulating questions that may make the encounter more interesting for both parties. The technique of repeating the examiner's question to gain time is often irritating and should be avoided. Marks are gained for demonstrating factual knowledge and logical reasoning rather than quoting endless lists of papers which may not be entirely relevant.

If the question is not clear, candidates should not hesitate to clarify the point. It is difficult, though not impossible, for candidates to change tack once they have started answering the question and realize that they are on the wrong course; though they should not change their opinions too readily. Candidates should not be evasive in their answers. If they do not know the answer it is sensible for them to say so, in order that the examiners can move on to the next question. Sometimes candidates have a tendency to be over-inclusive, especially if they know the answer very well. They should try to avoid showing off. If they are interrupted in full flow they should not feel upset. This may indicate that the examiner is satisfied with their response and wants to move on to something different. Candidates should not get into an argument with the examiners and should not lose their temper. They should try to give the information readily and voluntarily, rather than have the examiner do all the work in dragging it out of them. It pays to be polite but not obsequious, honest but not bullying, and warm but not over-powering.

Candidates should try to get into the spirit of the examination. After all, it is stressful for the examiners as well, and the easier the candidate makes it for them to get information from them, the more likely they are to pass.

References

Bhugra, D. (1990) *SAQs in Psychiatry*, Butterworth-Heinemann, Oxford
Holden, N. (1987) *Examination techniques in Psychiatry*, Hodder and Stoughton, London
Institute of Psychiatry (1975) *Notes on Eliciting and Recording Clinical Information*, Oxford University Press, Oxford
The Royal College of Psychiatrists (n.d.) *General Information and Regulations for the MRCPsych Examinations*, Royal College of Psychiatrists, London

2 Oral examination

General Principles

As noted in the previous chapter, it is vital in any examination to attend closely to the questions. Candidates should listen to *everything* the examiners say, but with an ear for keywords (see below). It is easy, especially when anxious, to seize on one part of the question and to begin building an answer around it while an examiner is still speaking. Candidates who do this will neglect important parts of what is said. They might, for example, hear the phrase 'He complains of auditory hallucinations,' and think with relief: 'Aha! Schizophrenia!'. They will then begin running through their management plan with such anticipation that they miss the examiner saying 'On enquiry the hallucinations only occur when the patient is drifting off to sleep, and the main problem is low mood and early morning waking'.

The examiners will not be trying to misdirect candidates: so they should not misdirect themselves through anxiety or a desire to jump the gun.

Keywords

PMPs often contain information which might seem to be mere background but which often gives useful clues. It is worth developing an ear for these keywords, but they should be regarded as helpful hints rather than all-important. The examiners nearly always refer to the patient by age and sex ('a 57-year-old man'; 'a 16-year-old girl'). They often also give information about occupation, race, ethnicity, social class or marital status which can trigger off associations from the candidate's base of theoretical knowledge. For example, if the question is about a 45-year-old unemployed male journalist· referred with auditory hallucinations, the candidate is more likely to suspect alcoholic hallucinosis than in a 23-year-old female travel agent with the same symptoms. Likewise, anorexia nervosa will be higher on the candidate's list of differentials for symptoms of weight loss and amenorrhoea if the patient is a 16-year-old ballet student rather than a 50-year-old housewife.

While these 'demographic' keywords help in suggesting diagnoses, other keywords may relate to the mode of referral and the setting where the patient is seen, and may give hints about the correct line of management. Suppose, for example, the question is about a problem which seems straightforward and not immediately pressing, but the referring general practitioner is seeking an urgent assessment. Use of the word 'urgent' suggests that the main issue is not diagnosis but the source of the general practitioner's anxiety. Is there something that has not been mentioned which is worrying him or her? The approach therefore should include the twin tasks of allaying the general practitioner's anxiety and dealing appropriately with the problem.

Similarly, the approach to a problem may well differ if the patient is seen in a police station rather than in an out-patient clinic, although the diagnosis is the same: in the former case the management is more likely to involve the Mental Health Act and court reports. The phrase 'in a police cell' suggests that the candidate will need to slip into a forensic mode of assessment, and respond accordingly.

After practising some PMPs the candidate may come to recognize these and other keywords, but should not rely on them exclusively. They might unlock the door to the answer, but the candidate will still need to open the door and walk in.

Length

PMPs can vary considerably in length, from a two-sentence thumb-nail sketch to a paragraph or two of detail. The length of a PMP determines in large part the style of the response and the subsequent questioning. It is worth becoming familiar with examples of short and long questions and the responses that best fit them. The PMPs in this book are of varied length and the answers differ in structure.

Short PMPs

These inevitably give little information, so the first step in responding is to say that more would be needed. The request should be specific however, for it invites the examiners to respond: 'Further Information? Certainly. What kind? From whom? Why?'

There is usually enough information in the PMP for candidates to have some idea about the likely diagnosis. With minimal information it is best to cast the net wide and be over-inclusive in the differential, using the further information that is sought to eliminate possibilities. If the information provided is simply that a 50-year-old woman attends the clinic with anxiety and restlessness, then there is a long list of differentials to narrow down. It helps to think of broad categories first—for example, organic, psychotic, neurotic, addiction, personality—and use these headings to suggest further information to pursue. A distinction should be made between further information sought *from* the patient and that *about* the patient, and, in general, the former should be asked for first.

Thinking aloud, the candidate might answer something like this: 'Well these symptoms are both common and non-specific, so further information is needed to clarify matters. First I would like to ask about associated physical symptoms. Does the patient find it difficult to tolerate the heat? Does she have palpitations, or a tremor, or goitre? Such symptoms suggest an organic cause, such as thyrotoxicosis, which could be investigated further. Then I would like to know more about the phenomenology. Is she anxious *about* anything in particular? Are there associated phenomena, hallucinations perhaps, which have caused the anxiety? She would need a full history taken and mental state examination to clarify this. A social history would bring to light any possible precipitants, such as major life events, which might suggest a reactive anxiety neurosis. A drug history might reveal that she has run out of benzodi-azepines and her new general practitioner may be reluctant to prescribe more without specialist opinion. A history from her husband might reveal that she has been an anxious person all her life, and the reason for her attendance is *his* inability to cope since his retirement, suggesting that the diagnosis relates more to personality than illness.'

This response is perhaps too full, but indicates the kind of thinking that candidates might adopt in their initial answer to a short PMP. Usually after the reply the examiner will narrow the field with more information, telling the candidate for example that the complaints are new, are not associated with any physi-cal or psychotic symptoms, and there has been no recent change of medication, but she has recently seen the general practitioner requesting that he sign her off work, though he could find nothing wrong. The candidate is now being led in a particular direction and almost invited to concentrate on employment issues. The candidate might respond by saying that he or she would enquire about any recent change of job or new responsibility, and might wish to check with the patient's husband or company doctor.

In this way the interchange between the candidate and the examiner leads stepwise towards a diagnosis. If the candidate gets there quickly he or she can be confident of two things: first, he or she is doing well so far; and secondly, the questions will now turn to management. The examiner might say: 'Alright, let us assume she has an anxiety neurosis reactive to an increase in responsibility at work. How would you deal with it?' The response should then be similar to that for a long PMP where this information is presented initially.

Long PMPs

Again, it is important to listen to the *whole* PMP, with an ear for keywords. Candidates should not then irritate the examiner who has just spent two minutes setting out the problem by say-ing that they would like further information, unless they are confident they can explain what information they want and why they want it. Furthermore, an overinclusive differential will not be helpful, for it will lead the candidate to tell the examiners what the diagnosis is *not*. This can of course be a useful approach if the candidate is unsure how else to proceed. A candidate can gain time to think by saying something like: 'Well, this problem doesn't sound like a personality disorder as you told me it began in her forties, there is nothing in the history or physical examination to suggest an organic basis, and the mental state reveals nothing psychotic. I suppose that leaves the field of neurotic disorders since you told me she doesn't drink and is drug-free.'

In general, a long PMP will require a response in which the candidate should aim for a more specific diagnosis, produced earlier, and with a shorter differential. The questioning will then move earlier to matters of management, and this is where the detail presented in the PMP becomes relevant. For example, if the candidate knows that marital work is important for the condition in question, and has been told that the patient's spouse has already refused to see the psychiatrist or the general practitioner, he or she will gain few marks by saying, 'The best treatment is marital therapy,' without elaboration. The candidate could say instead: 'for this condition marital therapy is the best treatment, but is obviously impossible if the spouse won't attend. I would discuss this with the patient and consider writing to the spouse, but if this fails I would consider other options such as . . .'

The appropriate line of management will often be suggested by the details presented in the PMP, either directly or by exclusion. In planning management therefore, it is worth following the maxim that most of the information contained in the PMP serves a function. Some of it may be the examiners' idiosyncratic embellishment of a story— though it is usually possible to tell when this is so—but the rest is valuable information that should not be discarded without thinking.

Decision Trees

Practice with SAQs will help the candidate to develop decision trees for particular subjects. Constructing these is a useful revision exercise, and helps the candidate to order his or her thoughts so that he or she can construct coherent management plans. Example decision trees are included in some answers to the PMPs in this book, and readers are encouraged to study one example each of a short (p.24) and a long (p.42) PMP before proceeding to test themselves.

Management Issues

Even if the problem seems straightforward, candidates should run through some general headings covering the various aspects of management to ensure that they do not miss something obvious. The following list is a general guide:-

1. *Physical*—Investigations, drugs, electroconvulsive therapy (ECT)
2. *Psychological*—Individual, group, couple, family, analytic, cognitive, behavioural, supportive.
3. *Social*—Day centres, employers, Disablement Resettlement Officers, Social Services, housing departments, industrial therapy, sheltered workshops, support groups, family support groups, voluntary services, etc.
4. *Legal*—Mental Health Act, consent to treatment, court reports, confidentiality, testamentary capacity, etc.
5. *Setting*—In-patient, day-patient, out-patient, general practitioner liaison.

Marks can only be gained by stressing the importance of liaison in these various aspects of management. This applies both to members of the multidisciplinary team and to those beyond it. As noted in Chapter 1, the examiners are often keen to assess the candidate's ability to get on with other members of the team. The key person for many problems will be the general practitioner, and even if the candidate cannot identify a role for the general practitioner in the case at hand he or she can always say that the GP would of course be kept informed.

Legal Aspects and Prognosis

In discussing the legal aspects of management, candidates *must* know the relevant provisions of the Mental Health Act. Even though the examiners in general are advised to avoid specific Mental Health Act issues because different parts of the British Isles have different Acts, it is important for candidates to use whichever Act they are familiar with. Similarly, prognosis cannot be discussed without an adequate background theoretical knowledge. However, candidates who have got on to issues of prognosis have probably done well enough on assessment and management to have passed, at least for that particular PMP.

It should be remembered that textbooks usually present prognosis in general terms for the condition in question, but in the PMP, by the time candidates get on to prognosis they will have a lot of specific information about the patient, and the examiners will be keen to hear them take this into account in responding. For example, instead of saying simply: 'Schizophrenia generally carries a poor prognosis in cases where . . .' they could relate the general and the specific as follows: 'The prognosis of schizophrenia is generally said to be poor, with a third recovering completely, a third pursuing a relapsing and remitting course, and a third remaining chronically ill. This case has a relatively good prognosis, in that the symptoms presented acutely, had a prominent affective component, and resolved rapidly with treatment. In addition, the patient's premorbid personality appears well adjusted, he has a supportive but not over-involved family, and he seems likely to comply with medication.'

Ending

PMPs last, on average, seven and a half minutes. The end might seem to come abruptly, because the examiners will be keen to move the candidate on to the next PMP. Candidates should not be perturbed if they feel that they did not finish the first PMP before moving on: this usually means that they are doing well, and that the examiners wish to challenge them further.

When one PMP ends and the next begins they must switch quickly back to their initial mental stance, and not allow the first PMP's style or content to influence them unduly. Examiners usually alternate, and will have different styles and different PMPs to draw on, so candidates can be required to switch, in the space of a few seconds, from a short PMP on child psychiatry, presented briskly, to a laconic long PMP on the psychiatry of old age. Intrusive thoughts and doubts about the first PMP can easily trouble candidates even once it is over, so they should practice making this transition under pressure, to make sure they can successfully remove the first PMP from their working memory while tackling the second.

Case presentations

Case 1.1

The medical team requests a psychiatric assessment of a 62-year-old out-patient with a diagnosis of chronic renal failure. He was diagnosed as having diabetes in his early 50s, and had complied with medication. However, four years previously, his condition had deteriorated: he started to lose his vision and he had to have three toes amputated because of ischaemia. He had been on twice-weekly dialysis for three years, and there is little likelihood of him being offered a renal transplant. The referral was prompted by his wife's concern that in recent weeks he had been polishing his gun collection and on one occasion had said he wanted to 'go out with a bang.' The physician says that the patient was a successful banker and describes him as a rather crusty, irritable individual, whose physical condition is likely to continue to deteriorate.

Questions

1. What questions do you need to ask this patient?
2. How would you plan psychiatric care of the terminally ill?
3. What role does antidepressant treatment play in management of such cases?

Answers

1. Before asking any specific questions, the initial approach to this man needs to be tactful if he is to co-operate at all. Only after initial trust is established can probing questions begin. Where a depressive illness is suspected in patients, such as this man, who are chronically or terminally ill, the familiar somatic manifestations such as fatigue are difficult to disentangle from the effects of the physical illness and its treatment. It is, therefore, important to consider more fully the cognitive and affective manifestations of depression. Attention should be directed at the patient's understanding of his illness, its treatment and his prognosis. The illness's effect

on various aspects of his life should be clearly established, and not only in a negative way—not just 'what else does the illness stop you doing?', but, 'what do you still enjoy?' Exploring these descriptions and cognitions will give access to his emotional responses to his predicament. Does he feel angry? Does he blame anyone? Does he blame himself? Does he feel guilty for the burden he is placing on his wife? Is he grieving for the career he has lost or the retirement he will not enjoy? The most difficult questions relate to his view of the future. How long does he think he has left? Does he fear he will gradually suffer more pain? Does he take comfort from religious belief? Is he resigned, fatalistic, hopeless or defiant about his future? How much has he been thinking about ending his life? Has he made any plans?

Asking these questions will be difficult for both the patient and the psychiatrist, but it will bring out any readily corrected factual misunderstanding, will help the patient to feel understood, which may in itself be beneficial, and will offer a possible avenue for treatment approaches. It will also be essential to ask the patient what he believes his wife understands about and expects of his illness (and to ask her too), and whether they are able to discuss the future together. If they are not, catalyzing their discussion may be the most important intervention a psychiatrist can offer.

2. *Psychiatric care of the terminally ill.* In addition to all the potential organically-mediated psychological consequences of physical illness and its treatment, terminally ill patients are at high risk of depressive reactions which may amount to illness, which often go unrecognized and untreated (Feldman et al., 1987) and may lead to suicide or requests for assisted suicide. Other patients who have an illness, which though not strictly terminal, is chronic, irreversible and entails burdensome treatment, such as dialysis, are exposed to similar risks, and the suicide rate amongst dialysis patients is disturbingly high (Abram et al., 1971). Psychiatrists may help manage such conditions through either a consultation model, where they help assess and treat those patients identified by the referring physician or, perhaps more appropriately, a liaison model, where they work together with the physicians to lower the threshold for

recognition of psychological problems arising in terminal care, and to develop methods aimed at dealing with these problems at an early stage. In this respect, their main contribution will be to help make explicit what is often unsaid or unasked, and to help patients to ask difficult questions or express fears, as well as to identify treatable depressive illness, and to guide patients through their anticipatory grieving. They may also help with communication between patients and their families, and support groups for staff working in this difficult area are often welcomed.

Case 1.1 decision tree

3. *Treatment*. Physically ill patients are at greater risk of adverse unwanted effects or drug interactions when treated with antidepressant drugs than those in good health. Antidepressants should, therefore, be used with care. The threshold for their use should be higher, doses should be cautiously titrated upwards, and the new 5-HT re-uptake inhibitors, with a different side-effect profile, may have a greater part to play as first-line drugs than in the physically well. This does not mean, however, that a clear-cut depressive illness in the physically ill should go untreated for fear of adverse events. The value of psychological therapy in the treatment of cancer patients is currently the subject of study which has shown it to improve the quality of life (Moorey and Greer, 1989). These results suggest that psychotherapy generally may have an important part to play in the treatment of depression in terminal illness, particularly in view of the difficulties of drug treatment.

References

Abram, H.S. et al. (1971) Suicidal behaviour in chronic dialysis patients. *American Journal of Psychiatry*, **127**, 119–204

Feldman, E., Mayou, R., Hawton, K., Ardern, M. and Smith, E.B.D. (1987) Psychiatric disorder in medical inpatients. *Quarterly Journal of Medicine*, **63**, 405–412

Moorey, S. and Greer, S. (1989) *Psychological Therapy for Patients with Cancer: a New Approach*, Heinemann, Oxford

Case 1.2

A 6-year-old girl is brought to the out-patient clinic by her mother and maternal grandmother. The referral letter suggests that she has great difficulties being by herself and follows the mother all round the house, saying that she would leave her like her Daddy did. The parents got divorced six months previously in a very acrimonious manner. When the mother and child are shown into the office, the mother insists that her mother (the grandmother) joins them. The child then stands clutching her mother's hand. She is the youngest of four children and has always played within the vicinity of the mother. She had become especially clinging after her admission to a paediatric ward 18 months ago. Her milestones have been normal.

Questions

1. How would you proceed from here?
2. How would you evaluate the parent/child relationship?
3. Outline your management.
4. What is the impact of bereavement on children?

Answers

1. Assessment should cover the reason why the family is presenting now rather than previously, and the pattern of development of the child's clinging behaviour. The information given suggests a long-standing difficulty in separating from the mother, which may reflect an exclusively anxious temperament in the child or chronic anxiety in the mother: questions need to be asked to consider these possibilities. It is also possible that the child's clinging only became excessive following the hospitalization or the divorce: the temporal relationship between the development of the symptoms and these events should be explored.

   Separation anxiety of this sort is often accompanied by sleep disturbances and nightmares, and by frequent physical symptoms, such as headaches or abdominal pain, especially at times of anticipated separation. The initial enquiry should cover this area too. A report from the child's school will help clarify how she behaves when separated from her mother during the day, and careful interviewing of the child may reveal the unrealistic fear about harm befalling her mother, which is characteristic of the condition.

2. The mother's insistence on being accompanied by her own mother during the consultation suggests that anxiety on her part may play a role in her child's presentation. The mother

and daughter should be seen separately and then together to observe their interactions. An informant account from the grandmother may help establish the nature of the relationship between mother and child.

3. In planning any management, both mother and grandmother need to be involved and joint family sessions may need to be conducted. After some sessions it may be possible to involve only the mother, though initially it is the child who needs attention. Hospitalization is to be avoided. Medication has a very limited role to play.

4. Children often show similar patterns to adults in reaction to bereavement. Some children do not appear to grieve openly at all. The grief in children is characterized by sadness, irritability, crying, sleep disturbances, nightmares, general decrease in interest and poor school performance, and sometimes temper tantrums, enuresis and conduct disorder may emerge. The short-term nature of the grief pattern is affected by how the child's needs are met and how caring adults respond to the child.

Case 1.3

A 24-year-old male schizophrenic patient has been remanded in custody at the local prison for medical reports. He has been charged with criminal damage and assault on the police, having smashed a window in the local post office and fiercely resisting arrest when the police arrived. The prison doctor has requested a psychiatric assessment as a second opinion.

Questions

1. How would you proceed?
2. Would you consider admitting him as a voluntary patient?
3. Once he comes in as a voluntary patient he refuses treatment, saying that you are a tool of the police. How would you respond?
4. Outline your management plans.

Answers

1. The first step is to gather as much information as possible about his previous episodes of illness and recent reports using case notes, nursing information, social services reports, if these are available, and verbal reports from the prison doctor and the general practitioner. Then the patient should be seen as soon as possible. During this visit further details of the circumstances of the offence can be obtained. The patient is interviewed to obtain his account of the offence and to assess his mental state at the time. In particular, his need for in-patient care should be considered, as should his risk to himself and others, and his understanding of the offence and his outlook. The aim is to get the patient out of the custodial setting as soon as possible, if he is actively psychotic at present, and to transfer him to a therapeutic environment. Choices include an immediate move to the hospital if he is in very urgent need of treatment, a hospital admission recommendation at his next court appearance (to either a locked or an open ward), or an out-patient hospital disposal at his next court appearance as a condition of probation. A hospital remand for further assessment is unnecessary if he is already well-known to the services. The multidisciplinary team should be involved in the discussion and, if possible, a nursing colleague should attend. The appropriate section of the Mental Health Act will need to be invoked, and practical arrangements for admission would need to be made.
2. Since he is already in custody, the courts will decide on the method of disposal, which may include voluntary transfer to hospital.
3. If he refuses treatment as a voluntary patient, he will be treated as any other patient and, if need be, appropriate sections of the Mental Health Act can be applied. The details of his mental state and behaviour at the time of his offence may be used to justify detention under the Mental Health Act, even if formal charges have been dropped.
4. If the previous diagnosis of schizophrenia is unchanged and the information from his previous psychiatric contact is available, he would need to be treated with appropriate

neuroleptics. Whichever drug he had responded to in the past would be the drug of choice. Appropriate doses should be given, for example, beginning with haloperidol 5 mg three times daily and then increasing the dose according to the response. At the same time, a psychosocial assessment needs to be carried out so that psychosocial aspects of management can be implemented, involving occupational therapy, family work, and rehabilitation services, as appropriate.

Case 1.4

The probation service requests a psychiatric assessment of a 46-year-old woman charged with shoplifting four cans of tomatoes from the local supermarket. The probation officer says that the woman has been remanded on bail for social and medical reports, having been charged with theft. When she was stopped by the store detectives, the woman burst into tears and said that it was her husband's fault.

Questions

1. What questions do you need to ask the probation officer before you send the patient an appointment?
2. Outline your assessment of the patient.
3. What recommendations would you like to make to the courts?
4. How would you manage her?

Answers

1. The contents of the social enquiry report should be studied, if available. If not, a copy should be obtained before submitting a report to the courts. Exactly what it is that the probation officer requires should be clarified, particularly

whether it is assessment alone, or assessment followed by treatment, if appropriate.

2. Before starting the assessment, the patient should be informed that the information she gives could go into a report to the court and that this implies a different level of confidentiality from that usually found in the doctor/patient relationship. It would then be necessary to establish her account of the alleged offence, followed by a full psychiatric history and mental state examination. This would allow a judgement to be made about her mental state at the time of the offence, which could form the basis of the recommendation to the court; and about her current psychiatric diagnosis and need for treatment. Depression is the diagnosis most likely in this circumstance, and the assessment needs to consider its onset, severity, precipitating and maintaining factors, and any suicidal intent. It seems that this patient's marital relationship may be relevant to her presentation, and therefore her husband may need to be interviewed separately as well.

3. Depending upon the information available from the woman, her husband and other sources, a report will be submitted to the court. This will also outline appropriate disposal recommendations, such as a plan for multidisciplinary treatment and support in the community as an out-patient. The report needs to be in lay terms and should include some idea of prognosis, stating why other disposals may be less helpful to the patient.

4. Management will depend on the diagnosis and the causal factors identified, and will involve pharmacological and psychosocial elements. Unless there is evidence of serious suicidal intent requiring close observation, she will best be managed as an out-patient, seen frequently at first and then at increasing intervals if indicated. She should be started on an appropriate antidepressant, such as a tricyclic, amitriptyline or imipramine, or a newer antidepressant, such as fluoxetine, the dose building up over the course of the first week and then being adjusted according to her response.

If marital problems are a major precipitating or maintaining factor, then marital therapy will be indicated in addition to the antidepressants.

Case 2.1

A 58-year-old man is brought to the clinic. His son gives a history that he had been found wandering across a busy road. The patient denies this, saying he had no recollection of doing so and, in any case, at the time he had been in a different town staying with friends. He denies excess alcohol consumption and describes himself as a social drinker. At interview, he is awake and alert, fully orientated to time, place and person, but there is evidence of impairment of recent memory. According to his son, the patient had become more forgetful in the previous six months, and would occasionally leave the gas on unlit.

Questions

1. List your differential diagnosis, with reasons for and against.
2. What investigations would you carry out to confirm your diagnosis?
3. Outline your management.

Answers

1. *Differential diagnosis*. The presenting problem is a six-month history of impaired cognition of sufficient severity to pose some risk in a 58-year-old man. There are several possible causes which could broadly be classified into depressive pseudodementia, a dementing illness or a sub-acute confusional state. Favouring depressive pseudodementia is the fact that it is a common cause of amnesia in this age group, but going against it is the lack of associated mood disturbance, the fact that the patient's son and not the patient himself is complaining of forgetfulness and the evidence of confabulation, rather than 'don't know' answers. A sub-acute confusional state is less likely, but must be rigorously excluded because of its eminent treatability. Going against it is the lack of evidence of a physical illness or other organic

cause, the focal nature of the memory deficit, with preservation of conscious level, and a six-month course without evidence of fluctuations in severity.

An early-presenting dementia is perhaps the most likely diagnosis, favoured by the mode of presentation, preservation of clear consciousness and the confabulation. Alcohol-induced Korsakoff syndrome remains a possibility, despite the patient's denial, though there will usually be evidence from the history or examination to support this diagnosis. A rare possibility is transient global amnesia, but the six-month history would mitigate against this. Dementia is not in itself a diagnosis, and the nature of the dementia would need to be clarified further. The most likely possibilities are multi-infarct dementia or Alzheimer's disease.

2. *Investigations.* A thorough history is essential to clarify the presenting complaint and associated features. In this respect, the son's account is vital, particularly with regard to any past history of head injury, depression, alcohol abuse, physical illness or drug use. Mental state examination should seek to characterize and quantify, using a standardized instrument, such as the Mini Mental State Examination (MMSE) or the Cambridge Cognitive Examination (CAM-COG), the cognitive impairment, and also to exclude any associated mood disturbance. A physical examination for evidence of alcohol-related harm, cardiovascular abnormality, such as hypertension or carotid bruits or other illness is essential.

On the basis of this evidence, investigation should be directed at excluding or confirming any suspected organic cause. It should, therefore, encompass full blood count and erythrocyte sedimentation rate (ESR), biochemical screen, with liver function tests, B_{12} and folate levels, Venereal Disease Research Laboratory (VDRL) and thyroid function tests. A computerized tomography (CT) scan will be important to exclude space-occupying lesions in the brain, but absence of cerebral atrophy on the scan does not exclude a dementing illness. An EEG may be of value in confirming and localizing any cerebral pathology, but there is argument about the diagnostic yield of this procedure. A chest X-ray will help identify any underlying occult lung or cardiac disorder. Formal psychometry may further clarify the conclusions of clinical cognitive testing.

3. *Management.* The first step in management is to make a diagnosis. Investigation cannot confirm a diagnosis of dementia of the Alzheimer type (DAT), which is perhaps the most likely diagnosis in this case, but it can exclude many other rarer causes. The diagnosis of a probable or possible DAT can then be made on positive clinical grounds using all available information and applying the National Institute of Neurological and Communications Disorders and Stroke

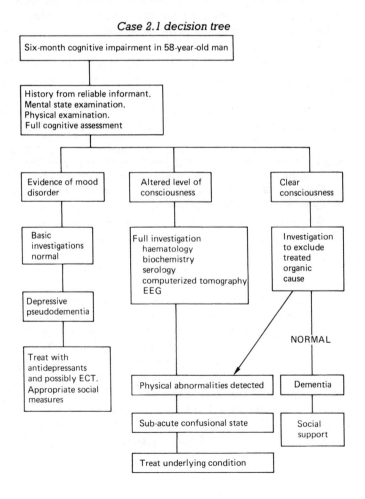

Case 2.1 decision tree

(NINCDS)/Alzheimer's Disease and Related Disorders Association (ADRDA) criteria (McKhann et al, 1984).

Assuming that no treatable alternative diagnosis is made, the emphasis is then on support of the patient and the patient's family at home, by minimizing the handicapping effect of the condition, treating associated physical morbidity and depression, and providing services, such as home help, meals-on-wheels, a laundry service, etc., with intermittent in-patient respite care, if necessary. The relatives should be involved throughout, and they will benefit from contact with local support groups, open discussion of legal issues, such as testamentary capacity, power of attorney and wills, and from discussion of the prognosis.

References

Folstein, M.F., Folstein, S.E. and McHugh, P.R. (1975) 'Minimental State'. A practical method for grading the cognitive state of patients for the clinician. *Journal of Psychiatric Research*, **12**, 189–198

McKhann, G., Drachman, D., Folstein, M., Katzman, R., Price, D. and Stadlan, G.M. (1984) Clinical diagnosis of Alzheimer's Disease: report of the *NINCDS–ADRDA* working group under the auspices of the Department of Health and Human Services task force on Alzheimer's Disease. *Neurology*, **34**, 939-944

Case 2.2

A couple have been referred for psychiatric assessment at the instigation of the male partner—an architect now aged 43 years. His complaint to the general practitioner had been 'we are not getting on'. The wife is a 42-year-old design consultant, and they have two sons aged 10 and 12 years, both away at boarding school. The couple state that their marriage was previously happy, but they have not been able to communicate with each other for about 18 months, since the wife discovered that her husband had had a brief affair with his secretary. She found her husband's lack of honesty shattering, and now feels that, since she cannot trust him any more, there is no point in trying to communicate.

Questions

1. How can you help this couple?
2. How would you assess their prognosis?
3. Describe the kind of work you would do in a typical session.

Answers

1. This couple present seeking help in returning their marital relationship to its previous happy condition, as opposed to continuing with the status quo, or accepting marital breakdown. Assuming the initial assessment reveals no psychiatric disorder in either partner, and they are both sufficiently motivated, marital or couple therapy is the appropriate treatment. This may be based on system theory, or conducted along analytic lines, or more commonly (and with better evidence of effect) through a behavioural approach. Whatever approach is adopted, initial assessment needs to consider the strengths and weaknesses of each partner, and of their relationship, and the way in which the relationship has changed over time. A behavioural approach requires each partner to identify elements of the other's behaviour they do not like, and to suggest, in specific terms, alternatives and the rewards they are prepared to offer for adopting those alternatives. A type of negotiation is therefore set up in which each partner 'gives to get', the aim being to establish a new equilibrium more attractive than the current status quo, by identifying and breaking the reinforcement of previously undesired behaviour. As with individual behavioural treatment, marital therapy should be time-limited (about 8–10 sessions), with defined goals, and an emphasis on 'assignments' between sessions, with reporting on lack of progress.
2. The fact that the marriage was previously stable, the lack of problems outside the context of the relationship, and the

apparent commitment of both partners to an effort to improve matters, all suggest a good prognosis, as does the fact that it is the errant husband who has made the approach for help. Outcome information is scanty but there is evidence that all forms of treatment are preferable to no treatment, and that the behavioural form leads to improvement in about 60% of cases (Gurman, Kristiern and Pinsof, 1986).

3. Lack of communication often becomes self-perpetuating. The husband presumably still feels guilty about his affair, and may seek to avoid his wife's accusing silence by staying late at work. This in turn becomes evidence for the wife of her husband's lack of interest in her. They could be encouraged to set up a bargain in which the husband agrees to come home at a specific time, and the wife reciprocates by welcoming him with a drink and an affectionate gesture. It is best if the couple arrive at such bargains themselves, but they will need prompting and encouragement to do so, and their subsequent progress in keeping to the bargain should be monitored at the next session.

Reference

Gurman, A.S., Kristiern, D.P., and Pinsof, W.M. (1986) Research on the process and outcome of marital and family therapy. In *Handbook of psychotherapy and behaviour change* (eds S. Garfield and A.E. Bergin), 3rd edn, Wiley, New York

Case 2.3

A 29-year-old Irish man has been admitted to the medical ward following a very serious overdose attempt. He had taken 50 tablets of aspirin, had left a suicide note and was discovered only accidentally. He says, amidst tears, that his boyfriend had died of AIDS six months previously and the relationship had been very positive and supportive. His family supported him during his bereavement and he subsequently discovered that his second HIV test was positive. He is a teacher and had been functioning reasonably well.

Questions

1. He wants to know more about AIDS dementia—what will you tell him?
2. What are the difficulties of treating somebody for depression who has AIDS?
3. What are the symptoms of ARC (AIDS-related complex) you will look out for?
4. What do you know about the 'worried well'?

Answers

1. Before jumping in with the prognosis of dementia, his degree of knowledge of AIDS should be ascertained; and how and when the diagnosis of his positive HIV status was made, the counselling offered, and his current status. If he has no signs of AIDS or ARC, it would be vital to find out why he has focused on only one area, whether he has any symptoms that worry him and also other associated factors. More details are needed about his suicide attempt. It will be important to bear in mind that in some cases this may not be the appropriate time to be discussing prognosis. Once his mental state has settled and more rapport has been established with him, various presentations of AIDS, including dementia should be discussed. AIDS-dementia complex develops over weeks to months and is characterized by motor symptoms as well as intellectual deterioration. A total of 40% percent of AIDS cases develop a neurological component and may have dementia, delusions or affective features. Typical early symptoms include impaired concentration, memory loss, mental slowing, apathy and agitation. Motor symptoms, such as weakness and poor co-ordination, may appear. Not all HIV positive cases will develop full AIDS and not all AIDS cases will go on to develop dementia.

2. The co-existence of depression and life-threatening illness is understandable. In addition, in this case, uncertainty about the diagnosis, perceived lack of social support and guilt over previous life-style may be contributing to depression. The difficulties in treating such a patient are similar to those faced with treating cancer patients. Moorey and Greer (1989) have described Adjuvant Psychological Therapy (APT) using a cognitive-behavioural model for managing anxiety and depression in such cases. The personal meaning of life-threatening illness can be considered at the levels of diagnosis, perceived control and a view of prognosis. The difficulties in managing such cases are particularly related to the patients who may feel helpless, hopeless, worthless and suicidal. Initial reports of treatment results are very encouraging. The aims of the treatment are to improve the quality of life by alleviating psychological distress and by inducing a fighting spirit. ECT (Schaerf et al, 1989) and cognitive therapy (Bhugra, Moorey and Minne, 1990) have been used successfully in patients where the terminal illness is AIDS. The patient's views of personal control, self-esteem and stigma of diagnosis can contribute to the difficulties.

3. ARC is best defined as symptomatic infection with HIV III in the absence of opportunistic infection or tumour (Weber and Pinching, 1986). To fulfil the diagnosis the patient requires one symptom, one sign and one laboratory anomaly. The symptoms include severe malaise, fatigue, lethargy, loss of more than 10% of body weight, unexplained diarrhoea for more than one month, fevers and night sweats. Signs include oral candidiasis, oral leucoplakia, persistent generalized lymphadenopathy, splenomegaly, eczema and folliculitis. A lymphopenia ($<1.5 \times 10^9/l$), thrombocytopenia ($<150 \times 10^9/l$), T-helper depletion ($<0.40 \times 10^9/l$), decreased lymphocyte nitrogen responses and anergy to 3 recall antigens (Weber and Pinching, 1986) are the laboratory anomalies.

4. The 'worried well' is a term applied to people in the community who may think without sufficient reason they have AIDS. They perceive themselves to be at high risk, irrespective of their proximity to high risk categories. They are worried about developing AIDS and they are well, in that they show

no objective signs of AIDS-related illness and are HIV nega-tive. They may present to the psychiatrist because they may have had bisexual experiences or occasional homosexual experiences, or may be psychologically vulnerable person-alities who may be responding to media coverage (Miller, 1986). They need to be assessed for psychological and func-tional disturbances because simple reassurance will not work. A discussion of their anxieties, assessment of their risk, dissemination of information and a confirmation of their understanding are important features in their management.

References

Bhugra, D., Moorey, S. and Minne, C. (1990) Cognitive therapy of AIDS. *American Journal of Psychiatry* **147**, 256.

Miller, D. (1986): The worried well. In *The Management of Aids Patients*, (eds D.Miller, J. Weber, and D.J. Green), MacMillan, Lon-don, pp. 169–174

Moorey, S. and Greer, S. (1989) *Psychological Therapy for Patients with Cancer*. Butterworth-Heinemann, Oxford.

Schaerf, F.W., Miller, R.R., Lipsey, J.R. et al. (1989) ECT for major depression in four patients infected with human immunodeficiency virus. *American Journal of Psychiatry* **146**, 782–784

Weber, J. and Pinching, J. (1986) The clinical management of AIDS and HTLV III infection. In *The Management of AIDS Patients*, (eds D. Miller, J. Weber and D.J. Green), MacMillan, London, pp.1–34.

Case 2.4

A 27-year-old woman wants help in coming off heroin. She has been 'chasing' up to 0.5 g daily for a year, and in recent months has begun injecting intermittently. She is frightened that she is putting herself at risk of HIV infection by sharing needles with friends, but cannot bring herself to use the local needle exchange programme because she used to work nearby and fears that she will be recognized.

Questions

1. How would you assess her drug use, and the risks to which it exposes her?
2. How would you manage her?
3. Would your management be different if she were pregnant?
4. What do you understand by the term 'harm minimization'?

Answers

1. The assessment should begin with an account of her current levels of drug use, by asking in detail about all drugs taken in the previous 24 hours, and average daily drug use in the previous month. For each drug, the amount, frequency, and route of use needs to be established, as does the occurrence of withdrawal symptoms before, or intoxication after, use. After this, a full drug history needs to be taken, covering all psychoactive drugs and alcohol; for each, her age at first use, her consumption pattern, and her reasons for moving to a different drug need to be established. Previous attempts at detoxification, whether conducted herself, or with medical help, need to be ascertained, with an indication of how long after each she remained drug-free, and why she resumed drug use. Risk assessment needs to cover her injecting practice and patterns of sexual relationships. Does she share needles frequently, or with many people? Does she attempt to clean them before use? Has she, or anyone in her circle, suffered hepatitis? Does she have sexual contact with drug users, and if so, do they share needles? Does she use condoms? Does she engage in sex-for-drugs transactions, or in prostitution to raise money for her drugs? Other aspects to consider include a medical and psychiatric history to assess any adverse affects of drug use, and a forensic history which may well provide a clue to her reason for presenting now, and her motivation for change. Has she been convicted of any drug-related offences? Is she facing any current charges, and, if so, is it likely that a court report will be required?

2. Her management would depend in part on the extent of previous attempts at treatment. If repeated previous out-patient detoxifications have failed, then a further attempt may well fail also; it would be better to consider referral to an in-patient detoxification unit. If, however, this is her first presentation, out-patient detoxification using oral methadone is the first line of management. Having established her current levels of drug use, she would be started on an equivalent daily dose of oral methadone. This will need to be dispensed daily by a chemist who has indicated willingness to undertake dispensing duties. The initial aim would be to avoid any further injecting, and then to gradually reduce the methadone dose over an agreed period to zero. Urine drug screens taken during this time will allow detection of any 'topping-up' with heroin, or use of other drugs. While she is engaged in detoxification, the opportunity should be taken to assess and deal with any additional problems underlying or complicating her drug use. These might include medical illnesses, housing problems, her receipt of social security benefits, and various psychological symptoms. She should be put in touch with drug users' support groups, such as Narcotics Anonymous, who can help support her through her detoxification and in her subsequent efforts to remain drug-free. It may also be helpful to mobilize support among her friends and family, and in particular to help her avoid contact with current drug users while she is withdrawing.

3. Yes, her management would be different if she were pregnant. Management of pregnant drug users requires close liaison between obstetric and paediatric services, drug dependence units and social services, to maximize the support given during pregnancy to the mother, and to minimize the risk to the fetus. Pregnant drug users may well be more motivated to discontinue drug use than previously, partly through concern for their child's health, and partly through fear that if they do not become abstinent their child will be taken into care. Women who present seeking help in this way should be reassured that drug use, in itself, is insufficient ground to take the child into care. Advantage should be taken of this motivation to undertake a planned, slow, detoxification during the middle trimester of pregnancy, to

reduce the risk of intrauterine growth retardation, prematurity, and obstetric complications associated with drug use during pregnancy. Sudden withdrawal should be avoided, as should detoxification in the 4–6 weeks before birth; the former may precipitate intrauterine death, and the latter premature labour. If abstinence is not achieved before delivery, the mother may require additional opiates during labour for analgesia, and the child will need careful observation by the paediatrician for withdrawal symptoms such as irritability and convulsions. After delivery, but before discharge, a plan of continuing support must be set up which adequately meets the needs of both mother and child and which will involve social services, the general practitioner, health visitors and drug dependence units staff. HIV positive pregnant drug users require particularly careful management to minimize the risk of transmission to the child and labour ward staff during delivery, and to maintain the mother's health throughout her pregnancy. For pregnant women who continue to indulge in practices such as needle sharing which put them at risk of HIV infection, the principal aim in treatment should be to reduce such risks as close to zero as possible.

4. Harm minimization is the name given to a pragmatic general approach in the management of drug dependent patients where the primary aim is not necessarily to maintain and achieve abstinence, but to keep the risks of exposure to adverse consequences of drug use as low as possible (Strang and Farrell, 1992). The rise of HIV infection in injecting drug users has led to resumption, in recent years, of this approach, which was originally developed in the more liberal era of the 1960s, but then fell into abeyance. The emphasis is on helping patients to avoid the most risky aspects of drug use, such as sharing needles, by providing needle exchange services and condoms, by giving advice on where to buy and how to disinfect injecting equipment, by prescribing opiates, sometimes even in injectable form, without a requirement that the patient move rapidly towards abstinence. Although the need to reduce the risk of HIV spread is the main driving force behind the practice of harm minimization, the same principles apply to minimizing the

risk of hepatitis B infection and accidental overdose. Throughout, the acceptance of a 'second best' option, rather than abstinence, need not imply that drug use is condoned. In exactly the same way, we do not condone continued smoking in a cardiac patient who has halved his tobacco use, but we praise him for his success so far and encourage continued efforts at reduction.

References

Department of Health, Scottish Office, Welsh Office Drug Misuse and Dependence (1991) *Guidelines on Clinical Management*. HMSO, London

Strang, J. and Farrell, M. (1992) Harm minimisation for drug misusers. *British Medical Journal*, **304**; 1127–1128

Case 3.1

A domiciliary visit is paid on an 18-year-old white man. According to his family, he was well until several weeks previously when he became suspicious, and started staying up late in his room playing loud music. He wandered around talking to himself and on one occasion, without provocation, was heard to shout, 'Stay away from me, you two', although there was nobody near him. His thoughts centred on his former warehouse job, and he claims he was persecuted by the police there. He was noticed at times to walk in a very odd manner. On one occasion he disappeared from home and was found by the police wandering aimlessly in a nearby park. He has not been eating well, and has not washed or changed his clothes in three weeks.

Both parents had previous marriages. A half sister, from his father's first marriage, was diagnosed as having an affective illness. The patient was born prematurely, walked at two years of age, and was delayed in developing speech. He was a shy, sensitive child, who left school at 16 years of age without any qualifications. Examination by an educational psychologist, before he left school, found him to have an IQ of 62.

On examination, he is found sitting in his pyjamas. He makes no eye contact and maintains a frozen expression. Waxy flexibility could be demonstrated until, when questions are directed at him, he begins to walk around aimlessly without responding. He says enough at one point to indicate that he is disorientated to time and place.

Questions

1. What is your differential diagnosis?
2. How would you confirm it?
3. How would you manage this case if he refuses to come to hospital?
4. What is the relationship between mental handicap and mental illness?

Answers

1. The patient seems to have a florid psychotic illness, with evidence of movement disorder, persecutory delusions, hallucinations and poor self-care, superimposed on a background of a family history of affective disorder and a mild mental handicap. Overall, the presenting features suggest a first episode of schizophrenia. But, given the family history, he may have an atypical affective psychosis, modified by the pathoplastic effect of his mental handicap. A drug-induced psychosis is possible and needs to be excluded. Epilepsy is common in association with mental handicap and a schizophreniform psychosis associated with unobserved seizures, or, alternatively, complex partial seizures in status epilepticus should be considered, though neither option seems very likely.

2. He needs admission to hospital for a period of in-patient observation and investigation, while a complete history is constructed from all available sources. He should have a urine drug screen to exclude a drug-induced psychosis, an EEG to exclude epilepsy, and a CT scan to exclude a structural brain lesion which might explain both his mental handicap and his current psychosis. His half sister's medical records should be reviewed for evidence of common features. Once he has improved sufficiently for testing, formal psychometry to quantify his mental handicap and to test for any focal cognitive deficits should be conducted. Finally, chromosome analysis for the fragile X syndrome might be of value.

3. Full investigation can only be conducted as an in-patient, so, if he refuses admission, use of the Mental Health Act should be considered. There is not, at present, much evidence of a risk to other persons, nor of immediate risk to himself, so it may be difficult to justify an admission under Section, especially if his parents are reluctant. In such circumstances, the best alternative would be to try to persuade him to take some medication and arrange to review him and his family again, giving them time to reconsider. It will be important to inform his general practitioner of this plan, as the general practitioner's knowledge of the family may help him or her

persuade the patient to accept admission. If, on review, he still declines admission and a section cannot be justified, or is objected to by the parents, then it will be appropriate to ask a community psychiatric nurse to visit regularly to support the family and to continue efforts at admission.

4. It is generally accepted that all mental illness is much more common in those with mental handicap than in those with normal intelligence. Approximately 30–60% of mentally

Case 3.1 decision tree

18-year-old man with mild handicap and florid psychotic symptoms

Needs admission for assessment
history, mental state, neurological examination
urine drug screen
blood tests, CT, EEG
chromosome analysis

DECLINES

Admit under Section

Schizophrenia

Affective psychosis

Drug-induced psychosis

Consider Mental Health Act

NOT JUSTIFIED

Continue persuasion.
Involve general practitioner and psychiatric nurse.
Symptomatic treatment with medication.
Attempt home assessment

Treat as patient of normal intelligence

handicapped patients have a diagnosable psychiatric disorder. In many cases, this is a transient behavioural disturbance or psychotic reaction not amounting to schizophrenia, but schizophrenia occurs in 3–6%, manic depressive psychosis in 1–6%, and neurosis in 10–15% (Reid, 1982). Although the classification of mental illness is not different in the mentally handicapped, the manifestations of individual syndromes are modified by the handicap. Handicapped patients may not be able to describe their hallucinatory experiences, and delusions may be incompletely formed or difficult to elicit. Diagnosis relies more on observation of behaviour than in those of normal intelligence, and requires more inference from observed behaviour to subjective experience. Drug treatment of mental illness is broadly the same in the mentally handicapped, but the place of psychotherapy is clearly limited. There is more scope for behavioural regimes, but these and drug treatments both raise issues of informed consent, which may not apply in the same way to a person of normal intelligence.

Reference

Reid, A.H. (1982) *The Psychiatry of Mental Handicap,* Blackwell Scientific Publications, Oxford

Case 3.2

A 40-year-old manic depressive woman, who has been symptom-free on lithium, wants to stop taking the lithium because she is putting on weight. She had her last admission seven years ago and has been symptom-free since then.

Questions

1. How would you advise her?
2. What other drugs can you use?

3. She tells you that when on carbamazepine previously she had a miscarriage and does not want to take it. She wants to sue the previous doctor because she has read somewhere that carbamazepine can induce abortions. How would you advise her?
4. Having decided that she should come off lithium, how would you proceed?

Answers

1. Before giving any advice, details are needed of the severity and frequency of her previous episodes, and the stability of her mood since she started taking lithium. In addition, it is important to assess the course of her weight gain before attributing it to lithium. She may, for example, have hypothyroidism requiring treatment in its own right. Once all this information is available, the pros and cons of stopping lithium need to be fully discussed with her.

   If it is clear that lithium is implicated in increasing her weight, that she has been euthymic since her last admission, and her episodes were neither very frequent nor severe, she should be advised that withdrawing it now is worth a trial. If, before starting lithium, her episodes were frequent and/or severe and she has had mood swings since, she should be cautioned against it. If she insists, it should be suggested that a compromise be made of taking a lower amount of lithium and keeping the situation under regular review.

2. The anticonvulsant carbamazepine has recently been licensed for use in the prophylaxis of manic depressive illness where lithium is ineffective or contraindicated, particularly where the illness is rapidly cycling. Another anticonvulsant, sodium valproate, is used occasionally although it is not specifically licensed for this purpose. In cases of recurrent manic episodes, antipsychotic drugs may have a prophylactic effect.

3. It should first be made clear that only medical advice can be given. For advice about suing her previous doctor, she should see a lawyer. She should be informed that although

the British National Formulary indicates that carbamazepine has a teratogenic potential, the risk is said to be small, while rates of spontaneous abortions at all ages are sufficient for it to be unlikely that carbamazepine was the cause in her case.

4. It is not yet clear whether lithium can be stopped abruptly or needs gradual reduction. It is best therefore to be cautious and withdraw it gradually over a month or two, and to see the patient regularly during the withdrawal period and for several months thereafter. It is important to offer the patient, her family and her general practitioner ready access to an early appointment as soon as she shows any symptoms suggestive of relapse.

Case 3.3

A 32-year-old man, who lives alone and is unaccompanied, is admitted to the ward with a history of depression. According to the notes made by the admitting doctor, the patient's parents and 24-year-old younger sister died in a car accident two weeks previously. The notes suggest that the patient had a very ambivalent relationship with his parents. The duty doctor noted that the patient had looked dishevelled and complained of loss of appetite and weight. He had also noted multiple abdominal surgical scars, for which the patient was able to give only a vague explanation. There was no past history of psychiatric illness. The patient is found to be a white male with normal affect who shows no evidence of anxiety or agitation, though he becomes tearful when talking of his parents. He demonstrates anger when asked for more information about his parents—'Haven't I suffered enough?' he yells.

Questions

1. How would you assess him? Give your differential diagnosis.
2. Outline your management plans.

3. Would you like to describe psychoanalytic explanations of this behaviour?
4. What drugs would you use?

Answers

1. Since the patient presents with depressive symptoms shortly after the reported sudden violent death of his family members, the first diagnosis to be considered is a bereavement reaction, possibly complicated by a major depression. However several features do not fit: his normal affect at interview despite his dramatic story, his reaction to questioning and his multiple unexplained scars, all suggest the possibility of a Munchausen's syndrome with both physical and psychiatric presentations. Malingering is another possibility, but would only apply if he were consciously feigning symptoms to avoid a specific event or responsibility, and there is at present no evidence of this. Clarifying the diagnosis will involve a search for more information to confirm or refute his history; but if he is pressed for more information or the veracity of his story is challenged, he will probably discharge himself abruptly, only to present elsewhere.

    Some hospitals distribute details of patients like this, to aid in their identification, and it may be worth reviewing any recent notifications, or contacting local hospitals directly to see if he has been admitted elsewhere with a similar story. While this is going on, he should be discreetly observed to see whether there are any differences in his behaviour at times when he believes no one is watching.

2. Making a diagnosis is, as always, the first step in management, but for patients like this establishing a diagnosis carries implied accusations of deceit and time-wasting. It is not surprising that patients then leave, and can rarely be engaged in any form of treatment.

    However, making a diagnosis of Munchausen's syndrome may well spare the patient unnecessary and potentially harmful treatment for medical and psychiatric conditions they do not in fact suffer, and, if it is possible to arrive at a diagnosis without alienating the patient completely, there should at least be an attempt to establish rapport. Although Munchausen's syndrome is a profound disturbance of personality which would require the very prolonged treatment these patients cannot accept, there may be associated symptoms, particularly depression, which might benefit from short-term treatment in their own right.

3. Because these patients avoid treatment, and therefore research, little can be said with confidence about the causes of the abnormal behaviour so strikingly displayed by them. Blackwell (1968) has identified several main factors: an abnormal desire to be ill (shared with other conditions such as hysteria and hypochondriasis); psychopathic personality traits; a knowledge of medical matters gained from genuine ill health or from work in hospital; and a precipitating life event. In addition, there has been speculation about the extent to which patients are motivated by masochism, with surgical procedures acquiring a sexual symbolism, and by a need for simultaneous dependence upon, and hostility towards, parent figures such as doctors.

Several authors have recommended the setting up of a central registry to aid the identification of patients such as this, the aim being to avoid unnecessary surgery, and to learn more about the behaviour and background of those who present this way. Although they are usually permitted to take their own discharge, some authors have suggested they need compulsory in-patient treatment to prevent further self-harm, though this may be difficult to justify (for review see Bhugra, 1988).

4. Unless there are associated psychiatric problems, such as depression, no specific drug regime is indicated in such cases.

References

Bhugra, D. (1988) Psychiatric Munchausen's syndrome: literature review with case reports. *Acta Psychiatrica Scandinavica*, **77**, 497–503

Blackwell, B. (1968) The Munchausen's syndrome. *British Journal of Hospital Medicine*, **1**, 98–102

Case 3.4

A 30-year-old Sudanese man is referred to the out-patient clinic at the request of a gastroenterologist. He arrived in the UK two years ago as a political refugee. He had been involved in anti-government demonstrations in Sudan, and at one of the demonstrations three of his family members and two friends died in a shooting incident. He was later arrested and tortured extensively. He managed to escape, and after stopping in various countries finally settled here. For the first six months he kept to himself, and then complained of abdominal pains for which he has been investigated extensively without discovering any cause. When you see him, he acknowledges that he has problems getting to sleep, and has recurrent nightmares about his torture. He has lost 13 kg in weight and is petrified about going out because he is convinced 'they are following me'.

Questions

1. What other information would you need to reach a diagnosis?
2. How would you manage him?
3. What are the possible aetiological factors?
4. What is his prognosis?

Answers

1. Various diagnostic possibilities present themselves, including depression, prolonged bereavement, a paranoid psychosis, and post-traumatic stress disorder. Each of these could be aggravated by his cultural displacement and isolation, and any of them might present with somatic symptoms such as his abdominal pain. To distinguish between them, enquiries should be made into his current symptoms, especially their time course, and a mental state examination should be carried out. If his loss of weight and initial insomnia is accompanied by other biological symptoms (including early morning wakening, diurnal mood variation,

anorexia, fatigue, loss of libido, and psychomotor retardation), then a diagnosis of depression appears most likely. If he is persistently preoccupied by thoughts and memories of his family, and behaves in such way as to avoid confronting the reality of their death, then prolonged bereavement is a possibility, though it is unlikely given other features of the case. If his comment that 'they are following me' reflects a belief or system of beliefs of delusional intensity, rather than an over-valued idea which is understandable in his circumstances, then he is suffering from a paranoid psychosis whose nature needs to be established. His unexplained abdominal pain would qualify him for a diagnosis of somatoform pain disorder, though this would not improve the understanding of his condition or guide his treatment. Overall, the most likely diagnosis appears to be post-traumatic stress disorder, in that he has suffered a major trauma, which he now re-experiences in his nightmares, and his initial insomnia suggests increased arousal. Other features which would support the diagnosis, and which need to be asked about, include flashback experiences, his response to reminders or symbols of his trauma, any evidence of avoidance of stimuli associated with the trauma, or more generalized emotional numbing, and, finally, other evidence of increased arousal (such as an exaggerated startle response, or hyper-vigilance).

2. There is little evidence to suggest that one form of treatment is better than others. For torture survivors, like this patient, one approach uses a technique called testimony. Here the therapy starts with one or two preliminary sessions to be followed by a detailed reconstruction of the events during torture. In these sessions a tape recorder may be used to record the detailed history. The transcripts of the session form the start of the next session. A very precise written statement is prepared and worked through for accuracy. Thus, repeated rehearsal of the traumatic events leads to habituation to the distressing memories by preventing avoidance. The private pain of the torture is often linked up with feelings of guilt, so that the patient may feel that he has let others down. It is important to help the patient see he

does not carry individual responsibility for the fate that might have befallen others.

Antidepressants, such as dothiepin, may improve the sleep pattern and reduce intrusive reminders if taken in a single dose at night. Some of the 5-HT antidepressants and phenelzine have been used. Benzodiazepines should be avoided.

3. The aetiological factors at work in producing post-traumatic stress disorder include a complex interplay of the initial trauma, and the patient's pre-morbid personality and post-morbid social support. Individual psychological factors are also important, whether considered in an analytic frame-work, or, more recently, in a cognitive or information-processing model. In addition, individual biological factors relating to autonomic arousal, endorphin release, and the pituitary adrenal axis have all been implicated to some extent. Much more research is needed to untangle these various different elements, and to develop effective treatment.

4. Post-traumatic stress disorder can be roughly divided into an acute form arising after a relatively mild stressor, and a chronic form following severe trauma. Most of the acute cases resolve spontaneously, but outcome for the chronic cases is poorer. Several follow-up studies of World War II and Korean War soldiers have demonstrated the long-term persistence of symptoms, with only 30% recovering completely. Even in those who recover, there may be a tendency to relapse at times of subsequent losses or increased stress (Kinzie, 1989).

This patient has chronic symptoms, and is socially isolated, with continuing physical problems. All these features suggest a poor outlook if left untreated, and probably a partial response to treatment at best.

Reference

Kinzie, J.D. (1989) Post-traumatic Stress Disorder. In *Comprehensive Textbook of Psychiatry*, (eds H.I. Kaplan and B.J. Sadock), 4th edn. Williams and Wilkins, Baltimore, pp. 1000–1008.

Case 4.1

A 48-year-old woman is referred for assessment of a depressive illness, and future management. Her first depressive episode occurred at the age of 17 years, since when she has had episodes most years lasting up to six months. The present episode started three years ago, out of the blue. She lost her concentration, became less motivated generally and unable to do her household chores, which led to her feelings of hopelessness. She was full of ideas of low self-esteem and expressed feelings of guilt. She had serially received adequate dosages of amitriptyline, maprotiline, prothiaden, lithium, carbamezepine and imipramine. She was admitted for a period of six months, during which she showed some degree of improvement, but has since declined readmission, though she has been fully co-operative with medication.

She has a twin sister who has had depressive illness which was treated by her general practitioner, although she did not require admission. Two of her uncles suffered depression—one of whom needed electroconvulsive therapy (ECT) as an out-patient.

On examination, she has a smooth midline swelling in her neck. She is slightly dishevelled and appears sad. Her speech is somewhat slow, though appropriate. She complains of lack of energy and poor appetite. Her sleep is variable. She feels worthless and incurable, and feels that she has let her family down.

Questions

1. What further information (including investigation results) do you require and why?
2. How would you manage her?
3. What is the role of psychosurgery in such a case?
4. Give a few side-effects of tricyclic antidepressants.

Answers

1. Since the onset of the present episode dates back three years, the diagnosis appears to be resistant depression. In such cases, the diagnosis needs to be reviewed. Further information from the history should include the patient's personality, the quality of premorbid and current patterns of adaptation, difficulties in interpersonal relationships, emotional conflicts, and sexual, familial or social problems that may have played a part in initiating symptoms or may be active in their perpetuation. Physical investigations would include full blood screen, serum B_{12}, folate and especially T_4 and TSH in this case, since she has a goitre. Scott, Barker and Eccleston (1988) have suggested that nearly half of females with resistant depression have hypothyroid functioning. Depressive symptoms may be the earliest harbinger of some occult somatic disease, which should be considered here, even if the long history makes it unlikely.

2. After reviewing the diagnosis and physical investigations, the dose regimens of the previous courses of drug treatment are reconsidered, remembering the possibility of a therapeutic window effect. If these have been adequate, various further physical treatments can be used. The antidepressants can be changed from secondary to tertiary amines or vice versa. ECT may need to be considered even if there has been no response in the past. If that fails, chlorpromazine can be added, which slows hydroxylation. Flupenthixol can be added. Antidepressants can be switched to tetracyclics. Monoamine-oxidase inhibitors (MAOIs) can be added or used by themselves. L-tryptophan may help, although following its withdrawal (because of its association with eosinophilia-myalgic syndrome) it is only available on a named-patient basis in the UK. L-tri-iodothyronine is reported to be effective in enhancing the sensitivity of noradrenergic receptors. Lithium salts can be used to augment all these treatments. In addition, psychological approaches, such as individual interpretive or cognitive treatment, or family therapy, may also be suggested. Continuous narcosis and sleep deprivation may rarely be used. Psychosurgery is sometimes indicated.

3. Currently, psychosurgery is indicated in severe, intractable depression with disabling symptoms for at least two years, where extensive pharmacological, psychotherapeutic and social interventions and ECT have all failed. Absence of psychopathy and 'good' premorbid personality are good prognostic factors. No satisfactory controlled studies have been carried out. In several uncontrolled series the improvement rates were 70% for depressive disorders (Mitchell-Hegg, Kelly and Richardson, 1976). Various destructive techniques (including suction, radioactive implants, ultrasound and thermocoagulation) of stereotactically located areas have

Case 4.1 decision tree

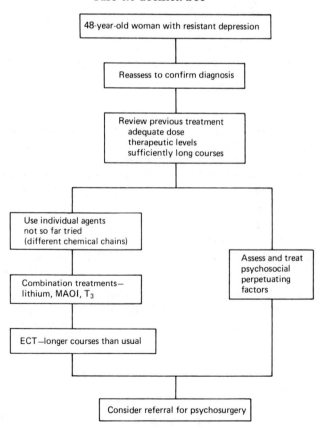

been employed. Appropriate post-operative rehabilitation is essential.

4. The side-effects of tricyclic antidepressants are numerous:

   (a) *Autonomic*: dry mouth, disturbance in accommodation, difficulty in micturition, constipation, postural hypotension, tachycardia, increased sweating.
   (b) *Psychiatric*: tiredness, insomnia, acute organic syndromes, precipitation of manic symptoms.
   (c) *Cardiovascular*: tachycardia, hypotension, suppression of ST and prolongation of QT and PR intervals on ECG, ventricular arrhythmias.
   (d) *Neurological*: fine tremor, incoordination, headache, muscle twitching, seizures.
   (e) *Others*: allergic skin rashes, cholestatic jaundice, agranulocytosis.

References

1. Mitchell-Heggs, N., Kelly, D. and Richardson, A. (1976) A stereotactic limbic leucotomy—a follow-up after 16 months. *British Journal of Psychiatry* **128**, 226–240
2. Scott, J., Barker, W. A. and Eccleston, D. (1988) The Newcastle chronic depression study: patient characteristics and factor associated with chronicity. *British Journal of Psychiatry* **152**, 28-33.

Case 4.2

A 23-year old student nurse attends the out-patient clinic at the request of her ward sister who has noticed that she spends a lot of time in the toilet and is suspicious that she may have bulimia nervosa.

Questions

1. How would you reach a diagnosis?

2. What kinds of therapeutic options are open to you?
3. Which would be your preferred option and why?
4. What is her prognosis?

Answers

1. It is possible that this patient has no psychological problems, and is attending only because her ward sister, through misplaced anxiety, has asked her to. In such a case it would be wrong to attempt any diagnosis, and it is more appropriate to address the sister's anxiety, involving, if necessary, the nursing tutor and occupational health department. Nonetheless, in view of possible denial of symptoms, and the sister's concern, a full assessment should be undertaken, comprising a detailed early history, general psychiatric history and physical and mental state examination, supplemented by information from an informant (such as a co-resident in the nurses' home), if one is available and the student nurse agrees to it.

   To establish a diagnosis of bulimia nervosa, it is necessary to demonstrate episodes of uncontrolled excessive eating ('bingeing' or 'gorging'), alternating with self-induced vomiting, or purging with laxatives, plus occasionally excessive exercise, in order to control weight. Patients may be of normal weight and continue to menstruate, in contrast to patients with anorexia nervosa, but may share with them an excessive concern about body shape and size. They will often show signs of repeated vomiting (pitted teeth, parotid enlargement, hypokalaemia).

2. Assuming the diagnosis is bulimia nervosa, the treatment options include:

   (a) Cognitive-behaviour therapy, in which the patient increases control over her eating by charting her food intake and urge to vomit or purge, so as to identify and address cues in the environment, whether external (e.g. particular shifts at work) or internal (mood changes).

   (b) Family therapy, whose value has been demonstrated for anorexia, but may be less applicable to bulimia nervosa.

   (c) Admission to an in-patient unit for careful supervision of eating patterns, along behavioural lines. This is best reserved for severe cases where other treatment has failed.

   (d) Antidepressant drugs, which treat the depression commonly associated with bulimia nervosa and may help by reducing the anxiety which underlies the urge to binge

3. For this patient, the first option should be tried initially, since it would be less disruptive of her training than admission, and because its main aim is to return to the patient a

Case 4.2 decision tree

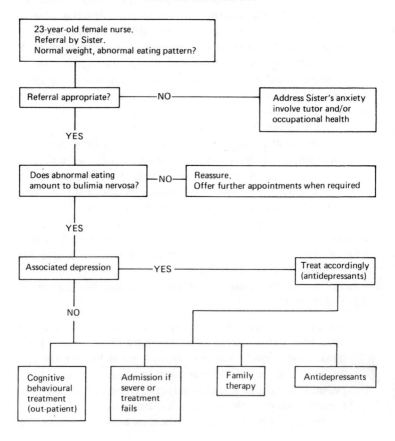

sense of control over her eating pattern, which should have a longer lasting effect than a course of drugs.

4. In describing it originally, Russell (1979) referred to bulimia nervosa as an 'ominous variant of anorexia nervosa', implying a poor prognosis with chronic symptoms and high mortality. Subsequent work suggests that if it arises without a previous episode of anorexia nervosa, the prognosis may be better. A distinction needs to be made however between abnormal eating behaviour and a full-blown eating disorder. The former is common, particularly in such settings as nursing homes and, in general, appears to be transient and not of special concern. The latter, being at the severe end of the spectrum, is relatively rare and likely to be persistent. It is likely, that while this patient may fall short of a diagnosis of bulimia nervosa, she might show some abnormal eating patterns: it should not be concluded that this in itself is associated with a poor outcome.

Reference

Russell, G.F.M. (1979) Bulimia nervosa: an ominous variant of anorexia nervosa. *Psychological Medicine*, **9**, 429–448

Case 4.3

A 68-year-old woman is seen on a domiciliary visit. The neighbours have been in touch with the general practitioner, who saw her and discovered that in the evenings her patient has 'visions', and she often stumbles around and has, on at least one occasion, sustained a fall.

Questions

1. What clues in the environment would you look for?

2. How would you differentiate between alcoholic hallucinosis, the hallucinations of delirium tremens, and hallucinosis unconnected with alcohol?
3. What other physical causes might you look for?
4. What would be your advice to the general practitioner?

Answers

1. Ataxia, falls and possible visual hallucinations in an elderly woman have a wide range of possible causes. The most likely possibility is alcohol abuse, which is not uncommon in the elderly, and an acute or sub-acute confusional state or delirium, which might arise from one of a large number of physical illnesses.

   Evidence around the house for the former might include: stores of empty bottles, a pervading smell of alcohol, signs of long-standing neglect, and, in the kitchen, cupboard and fridge contents suggesting a meagre diet of restricted range.

   There is less likely to be evidence favouring the latter in the environment, but it would be important to look for bottles of tablets, which might suggest a drug regime, or an already recognized but, so far, undetected physical illness. Evidence of incontinence, as suggested by a smell of urine or faecal soiling, could suggest perhaps a urinary tract infection or gastroenteritis, either of which could cause delirium.

2. Alcoholic hallucinosis is a relatively rare condition of uncertain status. The hallucinations are usually auditory and well organized, and arise in clear consciousness. Their content is often accusatory or insulting (which may lead to paranoid ideation). They are associated with long-standing alcohol dependence, possibly more often at times of relative increase or decline in alcohol intake, but are not limited to periods of alcohol withdrawal, as are the hallucinations of delirium tremens. These are usually visual, fragmented, and frightening in nature, and occur 48–72 hours after abrupt withdrawal of alcohol in alcohol-dependent drinkers, at

times of high autonomic arousal, agitation and disorientation. Visual hallucinations, unconnected with alcohol, generally indicate an organic illness, such as temporal lobe epilepsy in younger patients, or delirium in elderly patients, when there is usually an altered level of consciousness and disorientation.

3. There is a large number of possible physical causes of this patient's condition (Lishman, 1987). In an elderly woman, the common causes to be ruled out first include urinary tract and chest infection, drug reactions, cerebrovascular accidents, silent myocardial infarction and cardiac failure. If these are eliminated and a physical cause is still suspected, a search for progressively rare causes can begin, using appropriate investigation.

4. The home assessment, including physical examination, psychiatric history and mental state examination, may yield sufficient information to arrive at a confident diagnosis. If so, and if adequate home support is available from her family, neighbour and friends, or can be arranged without delay via the community services, then it would be best for her to remain at home while appropriate treatment is instituted. If home support is lacking, or her falls are sufficiently frequent to pose a risk, or there remains uncertainty about the diagnosis, then a short assessment admission is indicated. The aim would be to reach a diagnosis and institute treatment while community services (home help, meals-on-wheels, community nursing, etc.) can be set up. She could thereafter be followed-up via day-hospital attendances. Her general practitioner is likely to have a key role to play in setting up and co-ordinating community support, and taking responsibility for the medical aspects of her care while she remains at home.

Reference

Lishman, W.A. (1987) *Organic Psychiatry,* 2nd edn, Blackwell Scientific Publications, Oxford, p.130

Case 4.4

A 14-year-old adolescent girl from a council housing estate is brought for assesment. She is the youngest of seven children, and has been soiling herself. According to the mother, who is a rather poor historian, the patient has never been fully able to control her bowels. The reason she presents now is because the teachers in the special school that she attends have started complaining of the smell.

Questions

1. What would you do next?
2. How would you involve the family in the management?
3. Are there any drugs that you would use?
4. What is her long-term prognosis?

Answers

1. Initial assessment should cover the details of bowel habits. If the bowel motions are of normal or near-normal consistency, the most likely diagnosis is encopresis, while from the history it seems that it is primary or continuous, as there has not been one year of faecal continence. Alternative physical causes of soiling need to be excluded. If the motions are abnormal in quality: they might include inflammatory bowel disease, or chronic constipation with overflow leakage. If any such cause is suspected, a full physical examination is indicated to confirm it, followed by appropriate further investigation and treatment, which may involve referral to a paediatrician.

   Encopresis is associated with inadequate early toilet training and psychosocial stress. It would be important to enquire into the latter, since it is highly likely to be contributory in this case, given that the patient comes from a large family of low social class, and has intellectual impairment sufficient to require special schooling. If the mother proves too poor a historian, relevant information should be sought from other sources, including the father, responsible older siblings, school teachers, and their general practitioner. The aim should be to establish a full behavioural description of the child's bowel habits and to identify any unrevealed familial or social stresses which can then be attended to.

2. If the assessment indicates that unresolved family difficulties underlie the encopresis, these will need to be attended to directly, involving, where necessary, appropriate agencies such as social service, marriage guidance workers, the local housing department, and so on.

   The family will need to be mobilized in the treatment of the girl's encopresis by consistent, firm training, supplemented by such behavioural approaches as the use of star charts to reward improved control. This will clearly require sufficient involvement and motivation on their part, and they may need encouragement to persist.

3. Apart from using laxatives, if there is evidence of constipation, there are no drugs specific for encopresis. Some authors have suggested anxiolytics, but it is better to avoid drugs in treating adolescents with encopresis.

4. Encopresis has been divided into two types: regressive soiling, which is a return to an earlier stage of development following an upsetting event in the family; and aggressive soiling, which is associated with a poor relationship between the child and one of the parents, usually the mother, who is said to be excessively controlling and to have started toilet training early, thus bringing about the child's rebellion.

   The former type usually improves quickly as the child comes to terms with the precipitating event; but the latter is more persistent, especially if associated with faecal retention, in which case liaison with a paediatrician may be necessary. Whatever the cause, it is rare for encopresis to persist beyond the age of 15 or 16 years.

64

Case 5.1

Early one morning there is a call to the local police station to assess a 45-year-old divorced, unemployed journalist, who was taken into custody a couple of hours earlier for being drunk and disorderly. The police officer says that the patient has been 'talking to himself'; mumbling and lashing out in an agitated, fearful and angry manner. At times he appears terrified of imaginary objects. There is a previous history of drunk driving.

On examination, the patient is distressed, sweaty, tremulous, restless and agitated. He is unable to give a coherent history, but says that he lives alone. Occasionally he looks towards the corner of the room in a frightened manner, and on one occasion shouts: 'No, no, no. Just leave me alone.' He crouches, holding his head in his hands and weeps. He resists physical examination, but appears sweaty, has a marked tachycardia and looks pale with an old bruise over his right eye.

Questions

1. What would you do?
2. What is the relationship between alcoholic hallucinosis and schizophrenia?
3. How would you manage delirium tremens?
4. After this crisis is dealt with, how do you regard the prognosis of this case?

Answers

1. This man presents with atypical aggression and probable visual and auditory hallucinations in the context of alcohol consumption. There are no details of the amount he drinks, but there is circumstantial evidence suggestive of alcohol-related problems. Alcoholic hallucinosis and delirium tremens both present themselves as possibilities (the latter more likely), though concurrent diagnoses unrelated to

alcohol should be excluded. This case requires urgent admission to hospital for full assessment including a neurological assessment (in view of his old bruise), observation and treatment. He should not remain in the cell.

2. The central features of alcoholic hallucinosis include auditory hallucinations (second and third person) in a setting of clear consciousness, and unconfined to an acute withdrawal. In most cases it resolves spontaneously, but in others progresses to a schizophrenic illness. Cutting (1978) has argued that, while alcoholic hallucinosis does occur, it is rare, and that many patients to whom this diagnosis is ascribed, in fact have a psychotic depression or schizophrenia as well as heavy drinking. Kraepelin saw the condition as organically determined, and Bleuler as latent schizophrenic illness made manifest by alcohol.

3. In many centres, delirium tremens is regarded as a medical emergency, requiring admission to a medical ward. Wherever it is managed, essential elements in treating it include nursing in a quiet, well-lit room with monitoring of temperature, blood pressure, pulse and levels of consciousness. Adequate hydration (parenterally if necessary) is important, as is correction of electrolyte abnormalities and hypoglycaemia. Withdrawal symptoms require control with a reducing course of chlordiazepoxide, and large dose of B vitamins should be given to prevent the emergence of Korsakoff's syndrome. Where possible, these should be given orally, in view of anaphylaxis reported after injections of vitamins B and C (parentrovite).

4. Assuming that the current problems are related to long-term alcohol abuse, the first stage in dealing with them is to take a comprehensive history, when the patient can give it, supplemented by accounts from informants, and covering in detail the patient's drinking career. Any physical complications of alcoholism will need investigation and treatment, as would any underlying psychiatric disorder. Even after a thorough assessment and detoxification programme, if the patient remains unemployed and continues to live alone, he is unlikely to avoid further alcohol problems. He will need advice in deciding whether to abstain completely or to

Case 5.1 decision tree

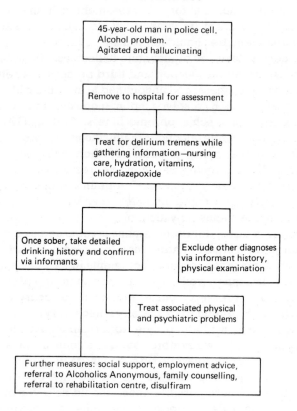

45-year-old man in police cell.
Alcohol problem.
Agitated and hallucinating

Remove to hospital for assessment

Treat for delirium tremens while
gathering information—nursing
care, hydration, vitamins,
chlordiazepoxide

Once sober, take detailed
drinking history and confirm
via informants

Exclude other diagnoses
via informant history,
physical examination

Treat associated physical
and psychiatric problems

Further measures: social support, employment advice,
referral to Alcoholics Anonymous, family counselling,
referral to rehabilitation centre, disulfiram

resort to controlled drinking. Referral to Alcoholics Anonymous may be of great value, and the prescription of
disulfiram (Antabuse), especially if his drinking is impulsive
in nature, may be a useful adjunct.

Reference

Cutting, J. (1978) A reappraisal of alcoholic psychoses. *Psychological
Medicine*, **8**, 285–295

Case 5.2

A 26-year-old single man of Jamaican ancestry is brought to the Accident and Emergency Department on Section 136, after being apprehended running around in the street, kicking at parked cars. Three days previously the patient had complained that he was 'possessed' by a number of spirits which were dominating his thoughts and actions. He admitted that the spirits were 'telling' him to kick cars. He had become restless and aggressive, with bizarre behaviour (e.g. running into his parents' bedroom when they were in bed and pulling away their bedclothes). He would step forward and backward in a repetitive fashion and would hold his arms in the air, as if in prayer, for long periods

He was six weeks premature at birth and was a poor scholastic achiever. He is still living at home, unemployed, and has few friends.

On examination, he is found to be a thin, tense, restless man who continuously paces around. He believes that he is the reincarnation of the singer Bob Marley, and admits that the thoughts in his head were controlled by spirits, as are the movements of his body. He says that he can hear the spirits talking to him.

Questions

1. How would you manage this patient?
2. What is his long-term prognosis, if the diagnosis is schizophrenia?
3. What are the common side-effects of neuroleptics?
4. What advice would you give the family in his further management?

Answers

1. This patient needs to be admitted for a full assessment, possibly under the assessment Section of the Mental Health Act. Since this appears to be his first contact with psychiatric

services, the purposes of admission are several, in that it would allow an opportunity to establish a diagnosis; monitor medication; form lasting relationships with the patient and his relatives; educate them; and to formulate a plan of social management. After admission, he would need to be observed drug-free. Drug-induced states, manic excitement and organic brain syndromes would need to be excluded before arriving at a diagnosis of schizophrenia. Appropriate medication, such as the sedating neuroleptic chlorpromazine, should then be started with titration of the dose, and the patient gradually initiated into ward activities, occupational therapy, etc. Multi-disciplinary assessment needs to be carried out.

2. Several features suggest a poor prognosis: social isolation, poor educational achievement, and unemployment. However, he demonstrates catatonic features which are a good prognostic sign, as is the apparently acute onset. The outcome is determined by other factors as well, including levels of Expressed Emotion within the family. There is evidence that high levels of hostility, critical comment, and over-involvement with a key relative, to whom the patient is exposed for more than 35 hours a week, are associated with increased relapse rates (Vaughn and Leff, 1976).

3. The neuroleptics (phenothiazines and butyrophenones) have the following side-effects:

    (a) Acute dyskinesia and dystonias,which are more common in younger males and include opisthotonos, tonic contractions of neck, mouth, tongue and postural muscles, and oculogyric crisis.
    (b) Extra-pyramidal side-effects include the Parkinsonian triad of bradykinesia, stiffness, and tremor, as well as akathisia.
    (c) Anticholinergic side effects, such as dry mouth, blurred vision, retention of urine, constipation, tachycardia, and postural hypotension.
    (d) Others, such as depression, weight gain, seizures, skin photosensitivity, blood dyscrasia, reduced libido, galactorrhoea, cholestatic jaundice, etc.

(e) Tardive dyskinesia and, rarely, neuroleptic malignant syndrome.

4. In the short-term, the principles of dealing with the family include:

   (a) appreciating their difficulties;
   (b) being realistic about their capabilities;
   (c) helping them come to a realistic understanding of the patient's condition and future prospects.

In the medium and long-term, educating relatives about the illness is extremely important, and this may take several sessions. The nature of the illness, its possible causation, the prognosis and effects of drugs, should be clearly explained in lay language. Specific difficulties should be gone into and explained. The relatives' knowledge and attitudes need to be explored. High levels of expressed emotion should be looked out for. The relatives should try to accept that the schizophrenic experiences are real to the patient and realistic limits need to be set on his behaviour. A degree of separation, through day-hospital or day-centre, may be helpful. Relatives' groups can be very useful in providing support and education. Voluntary agencies too can be very important in providing valuable support in the community.

Reference

Vaughn, C. and Leff, J.P. (1976) The influence of family and social factors on the course of schizophrenic illness. *British Journal of Psychiatry*, **129**, 125–137

Case 5.3

A 5-year-old boy is referred for psychiatric assessment with a history of habitual facial spasms. These started about a year ago but have increased dramatically within the last two months when he started school, and his parents separated at this time.

70

Questions

1. What is your differential diagnosis?
2. What is the general prognosis of tics?
3. List possible explanations of aetiological factors in this case.
4. What drugs would you use?

Answers

1. The most likely diagnosis is that the child suffers from tics. Tics are sudden involuntary repetitive purposeless movements of circumscribed groups of muscles.

   Tics need to be distinguished from less common but more serious abnormal movements, which are usually indicative of underlying neurological disorder. They include: choreiform movements, which are tic-like in nature but can involve any muscle groups; athetoid movements, which are slow and writhing and especially affect distal parts; dystonic movements, which are often well-localized but are slow and sustained; and myoclonic jerks which bring shock-like contractions. Although tics and choreiform movements are similar, and both cease in sleep, distinguishing them is aided by the lack of repetition in the latter, associated with hypotonia and incoordination.

2. Generally, the prognosis of tics is good. At least one half of cases recover over a five-year period and two thirds over eight years. Obsessional traits and development of coprolalia are bad prognostic features, as these suggest a diagnosis of Gilles de la Tourette syndrome. While transient tic-like symptoms are very common in children, they occur more frequently in boys, and are associated with other developmental disorders. Their onset is very commonly at the time of some emotional distress.

3. In this child, starting school and parental separation seem obvious precipitants. The general opinion is that tics are exaggerated motor responses to stress. The child is unable to tolerate a build up of tension and it overflows into useless motor activity.

4. There are no drugs specifically indicated unless associated coprolalia, suggesting Tourette's syndrome, is present, in which case haloperidol can be used. Some authors have recommended using anxiolytics to reduce tension, but great caution should be exercised in using these drugs in such an age group. A better approach involves trying to reduce the background stresses and dealing with the symptom using behavioural methods, such as relaxation exercises with bio-feedback, and massed practice.

Case 5.4

The general practitioner has requested an assessment of a 70-year-old widow who lives by herself. Her daughter, when visiting her over the weekend, discovered that her mother had been incontinent and the house had 'gone to seed'. She had been a very house-proud woman and had managed to cope very well with her husband's death some six years ago. The daughter is also worried that her mother may be demented.

Questions

1. What would you cover in your initial assessment?
2. What would be your main differential diagnosis?
3. What memory tests would you use?
4. After assessing her you discover that she is depressed. What would you do next?

Answers

1. More information is required from the general practitioner, especially regarding the previous medical history and medication. In her environment, the general level of cleanliness should be assessed, as should the state of repair of the house, heating, lighting, ventilation, water supply, the stairs,

possible accident hazards, empty bottles and other evidence of alcohol abuse. Her safety and mobility round the house need to be assessed, to determine whether the environment is suitable for her. A major advantage of a domiciliary visit is that the patient is being assessed in a familiar situation so her function in her own environment and her level of social support can be easily ascertained.

2. After excluding physical causes of incontinence, the main differential diagnosis lies between dementia, depressive pseudodementia, and delirium. A diagnosis of dementia is more likely if there is a long history, with memory deficits presenting first and gradually progressing in clear consciousness. A global impairment of cognitive function is definitive, and while it may vary in intensity, it will not remit. During testing, patients usually give incorrect, rather than 'don't know', answers, and they may display circumstantial and catastrophic reactions. Patients with depressive pseudodementia often have a past history or family history of depression, and may display associated affective symptoms. They are often aware of, and distressed by, their memory impairment, and, on testing, avoid answering more often than making mistakes. A delirium (i.e. acute or subacute confusional state) is likely to be marked by clouding of consciousness and fluctuations in severity, and may be suggested by associated physical findings, such as a fever.

Distinguishing these diagnoses, especially the first two, may be difficult and requires as full information as possible from the general practitioner, family, and friends, as well as physical and mental state examination. Even then, a therapeutic trial of antidepressants may be called for.

3. As well as standard clinical tests assessing temporospatial orientation, registration, short-term recall, long-term memory, and concentration, a variety of standardized tests yielding scores are available. The Abbreviated Mental Test of Hopkins is easily memorized, and the Mini-mental State (Folstein, Folstein and McHugh, 1975) is widely used. More detailed tests (such as the CAMCOG element of the Cambridge Mental Disorders of the Elderly Examination (CAMDEX) structured interviews for assessment of the elderly)

are available, and give more detailed information, but take longer, and are more arduous.

4. If the patient is depressed and needs to be treated and agrees to come in, it might be sensible to admit her for a short while. This has several advantages because it will enable her physical condition to be assessed thoroughly. She can also be commenced on antidepressants which, in the initial stages, may produce severe side-effects, such as postural hypotension, which may be a problem if she is living by herself. In addition, the risk of suicide needs to be considered in making this decision. If there is no family support

Case 5.4 decision tree

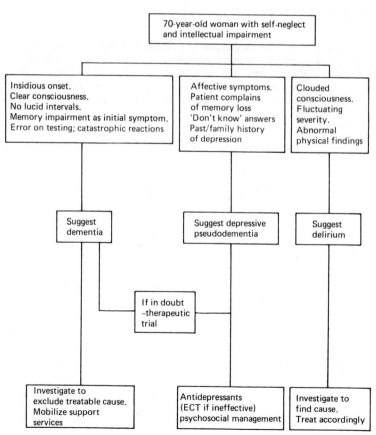

available, the patient refuses to come in, and suicidal risk is not serious, community support via the community psychiatric nurse and social worker will need to be arranged while treatment is commenced. The medication used should be an antidepressant with low side-effects, e.g. lofepramine, or one of the newer 5-HT antidepressants such as fluvoxamine, fluoxetine, or sertraline.

Concurrently with drug treatment, psychological approaches, such as guided mourning for her husband, and social management, such as day-centre referral, need to be undertaken.

References

Hopkins, H.M. (1972) Evaluation of a mental test score for assessment of mental impairment in the elderly. *Age and Ageing,* 1, 233–238.

Folstein, M.F., Folstein, S.E. and McHugh, P.R. (1975) 'Mini Mental State'. A practical method for grading the cognitive state of patients for the clinician. *Journal of Psychiatric Research,* 12, 189–198.

Case 6.1

A 50-year-old Spanish woman, who has been living in the UK for 30 years, is referred to the outpatient clinic with 'claustrophobia'. For many years, ever since she fainted and was incontinent in a lift, she has felt anxious and panicky at the prospect of using a lift again and prefers to take the stairs instead. In addition, she has avoided travel on the underground for several years, though she can travel by trains and buses. She recently refused promotion because it would have meant her having to take a lift up 11 floors every day. She admits to drinking wine with meals in the evenings almost every day. Her husband is increasingly disabled by arthritis.

On examination, she is well-dressed and mildly nervous. She denies depression, but feels constrained by her difficulties. There are no abnormal experiences, perceptions or behaviour.

Questions

1. What areas would you like to cover in your assessment?
2. What is the aetiology of phobic neurosis and how does it relate to treatment?
3. What is the most suitable treatment package for this case and what would you do?
4. What are the important predictors of treatment response?

Answers

1. The assessment should cover the exclusion of other psychiatric illness, such as depression, and physical illness. Depression may be the primary diagnosis, with phobic symptoms as one manifestation. A drug and alcohol history should indicate the degree to which the patient uses self-medication to reduce her anxiety. If no underlying causes are evident, the diagnosis is most likely to be a phobic anxiety neurosis (i.e. a disproportionate fear of a particular class

of objects or situation which is irrational and leads to avoidance). The motivation of the patient and the spouse to persist with treatment needs to be ascertained. A detailed account of the phobia, including the precise nature of the feared consequence, the circumstances in which it arises, the modifying factors, disruption to everyday life, etc., needs to be obtained and supplemented by information from her husband. The episode of incontinence needs to be assessed, in case there is evidence of epilepsy.

2. Psychoanalytic theory suggests that the feared object or situation is a symbolic representation of an anxiety arising from deep-seated conflicts, which is excluded from consciousness by the mechanisms of repression and displacement. Learning theory may account for a salient feature of the phobia, i.e. avoidance of the feared object, as a perpetuating feature, but has difficulty explaining the onset of the first episode of anxiety. Whatever the origin, the treatment is based on the premise that controlled gradual exposure to the feared stimulus will lead to progressive and sustained reduction of the fear.

3. She appears to have separate but similar fears of travelling in lifts and on underground trains. For each of these fears, a target of treatment should be identified in specific terms (e.g. taking the lift unaccompanied to a specified floor and back twice a day for a specified number of days) as well as a series of intermediate weekly targets of increasing difficulty, beginning with just standing in the stationary lift with her husband or other co-therapist. At each stage, the aim should be to remain in the anxiety-provoking situation for as long as it takes for the anxiety to subside, for the patient to monitor her level of anxiety before, during and after each period of exposure, and for the treatment to be repeated once or twice daily with as much help from the co-therapist as possible.

4. Without treatment, phobic responses can often persist for many years. The patient may respond by learning to co-exist with the condition by suitable adaptation of her lifestyle, by developing recurrent or prolonged episodes of depression or by maladaptive self-medication with drugs or alcohol.

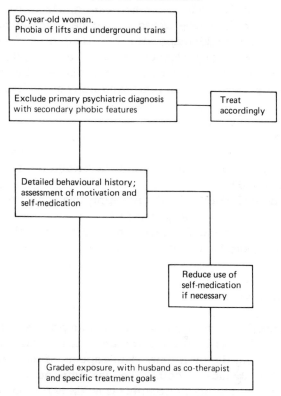

Case 6.1 decision tree

```
┌─────────────────────────────────────┐
│ 50-year-old woman.                   │
│ Phobia of lifts and underground trains│
└─────────────────────────────────────┘

┌─────────────────────────────────────┐      ┌──────────────┐
│ Exclude primary psychiatric diagnosis│──────│ Treat        │
│ with secondary phobic features       │      │ accordingly  │
└─────────────────────────────────────┘      └──────────────┘

┌─────────────────────────────────────┐
│ Detailed behavioural history;        │
│ assessment of motivation and         │
│ self-medication                      │
└─────────────────────────────────────┘

                        ┌──────────────┐
                        │ Reduce use of│
                        │ self-medication│
                        │ if necessary │
                        └──────────────┘

┌─────────────────────────────────────┐
│ Graded exposure, with husband as co-therapist│
│ and specific treatment goals         │
└─────────────────────────────────────┘
```

The most important single determinant of response to treatment is motivation. Patients can often be encouraged by a family member who is willing to act as a co-therapist and support their efforts. Behaviour therapy appears more effective for the more specific phobias. The presence of secondary gain is a bad prognostic sign.

Case 6.2

The casualty department requires an assessment of a 48-year-old vagrant who has been taken there by the police. The police say that he was shouting in the street and told them that he was frightened of the voices he was hearing. These came from behind him, but when he turned around there was no one there and the voices would temporarily stop. He gives a 30-year history of almost daily alcohol use, and acknowledges 'the shakes' most mornings, which he needs to relieve by drinking. He appears dishevelled and smells strongly of alcohol.

Questions

1. How would you assess him and what would be your initial management?
2. How does the Mental Health Act apply to alcohol problems?
3. How do you see his prognosis?
4. There is much media speculation about mental illness and the homeless. Summarize your view.

Answers

1. This man has evidence of long-standing alcohol dependence, and superimposed distressing auditory hallucinations of uncertain duration. Important aspects of the history to establish include: whether he has stopped drinking in recent days for any reason (this is unlikely because he still smells of drink); whether the hallucinations have arisen acutely or have been present for some time and whether there has been any intercurrent physical illness or head injury.

   Diagnostic possibilities include: alcoholic hallucinosis, delirium tremens brought on by alcohol withdrawal, or a delirious state caused by an underlying physical illness, such as a chest infection, or head injury incurred while drunk. He needs physical examination and initial investigation to rule out these latter possibilities, and he needs admission to hospital to complete his assessment and manage his condition. Once admitted, he needs alcohol detoxification, intensive vitamin replacement, and appropriate nursing care. Any underlying physical illness detected will need to be treated, and alcoholic hallucinosis may need specific treatment with anti-psychotic agents.

2. For the purposes of the Mental Health Act 1983, dependence on alcohol or drugs is not regarded as 'a mental disorder' for the treatment of which a patient may be committed to hospital. Furthermore, a purely physical illness arising from alcohol abuse, such as alcoholic gastritis, is also not considered a cause for compulsory admission to hospital for treatment. However, if alcohol dependence is associated with another mental disorder, such as delirium tremens or alcoholic hallucinosis or alcohol-induced depressive illness, then these secondary mental disorders may be grounds for compulsory admission to hospital for treatment. It would then be appropriate to treat the underlying dependence, in so far as the patient consents, and for so long as the terms of the original section continue to apply.

   In these circumstances, where the diagnosis is in some doubt, but where there is evidence of a delirium or psychosis associated with alcohol dependence, the appropriate section to use would be a Section 2 (in England and Wales), permitting a one month period of assessment and initial treatment. If, after initial treatment, the psychosis or delirium clears completely, but the patient displays no wish to undergo treatment of his underlying alcohol dependence, the section should be rescinded, and he should be allowed to leave.

3. This man's age, his long history, his homelessness, his lack of social support, and his presumed physical frailty, all combine to suggest a very poor prognosis. This does not mean that he is not worthy of treatment, however, and he should be offered as vigorous an attempt at detoxification as anyone else. A number of voluntary agencies exist to help patients in this group, including alcohol detoxification hostels and treatment centres for alcoholics. Enough patients with very poor prognoses confound their doctor's pessimism to make these options worth a try.

4. Whilst it is likely that in historical terms the homeless have always had high rates of alcoholism and other mental disorder, the rapid expansion of asylums from the Victorian era until the post-war years, removed many of these patients

from the public view. The closure of the asylums, and their replacement by insufficient numbers of community care facilities, from which patients lose contact all too easily, has returned many of them to the streets and to public awareness, though some studies have not confirmed this. In addition, they have been joined by a younger group, moving to large cities for economic reasons, but unable to find housing or work there. This group displays significant levels of alcohol abuse, but not necessarily dependence, together with drug taking and consequent psychiatric problems. Finally, there are 'the new chronic' cases of schizophrenia and other major mental illness, whose initial breakdowns prove resistant to treatment, and who drift away from their families and from hostel and group home accommodation to roam the streets in a floridly psychotic state. It should not be assumed that psychiatric illness in the homeless is an homogeneous problem, and any attempts to deal with it must address these various subgroups appropriately.

Case 6.3

A 52-year-old woman is brought to the clinic by a worker from the hostel where she had been resident for 10 years or so. She had previously spent many years in a mental hospital, carrying a diagnosis of schizophrenia, and treated with chlorpromazine. During her time in the hostel, she had been well-settled and happy, but one month previously, she was noted to make chewing and sucking movements of her mouth and lips, and occasionally would smack her lips loudly. These movements did not appear to cause her distress, but other residents and staff repeatedly commented upon them and asked her to stop, causing some tension in the hostel. The hostel would like to discuss the cause of these movements, and what can be done about them.

Questions

1. What advice would you give?
2. What are the predisposing factors for this condition?
3. What is the best way of dealing with this problem?

Answers

1. It is likely that the patient has developed tardive dyskinesia, caused by her long-term neuroleptic treatment. It manifests itself in involuntary movements, commonly affecting the tongue, lips and neck, but also, on occasions, involving the extremities and abnormalities of posture, especially in younger patients. Although it is not in itself life-threatening or painful, the condition can cause considerable distress to the patient and others, as seems to be happening in this case. Although it is relatively common in those treated with long-term neuroleptics, with a prevalence of some 15%–20% in this group, it is in many cases mild and only infrequently severe. It is likely to continue long-term, although in some cases the symptoms will gradually fade over a period of months following changes to the drug regime. The hostel worker should be told that although chlorpromazine may well have caused the symptoms, withdrawing it at this stage is likely to make them worse, at least in the short-term. There are other ways of providing some symptomatic benefit (see below).
2. The clearest risk factor for tardive dyskinesia is long-term treatment with any neuroleptic. Estimates suggest an accumulative incidence of 3% per year, at least for the first few years of neuroleptic treatment. The risk rises with increasing age, but so does the risk of tardive dyskinesia-like syndrome in the absence of neuroleptic treatment. Women appear to be more at risk than men, particularly in older age groups. It does not appear to be particularly associated with one neuroleptic or one group of agents. The risk appears to rise with increasing dose of neuroleptics and with duration of treatment.

3. Once the condition has developed, it is commonly irreversible and treatment is difficult. Withdrawing the putative causal drug commonly makes symptoms worse. They can be suppressed by increasing the dose of the drug, or adding another anti-psychotic agent. It is uncertain whether this merely delays the emergence of symptoms, or actually aggravates them in the long-term. Anti-Parkinsonian agents generally make the condition worse, and should not be used. Amine-depleting drugs, such as reserpine and tetrabenazine, may be of benefit, as may cholinergic agents, such as physostigmine.

On the whole, it is much better to prevent the condition arising by being very thorough about initial diagnosis, by using drugs in the lowest effective dose, and by considering the use of 'drug holidays', although it is still unclear whether such 'drug holidays' reduce the long-term risk of tardive dyskinesia, or simply make it easier to diagnose the condition early on. Pharmacological research is still trying to identify anti-psychotic agents which have a reduced risk of extra-pyramidal effects, in general, and tardive dyskinesia, in particular, and one such is clozapine, though this carries other serious risks like agranulocytosis.

The decision to use neuroleptics therefore requires a judgement about the balance between the benefit afforded any individual patient, and the long-term risk of tardive dyskinesia developing. Malpractice litigation in the USA has made it commonplace for patients to be informed of the risks of tardive dyskinesia before treatment there, and although this may not be standard practice in the UK, it is difficult to justify not informing patients.

Case 6.4

A husband and wife attend the clinic seeking advice about starting a family. The husband is a 28-year-old plumber, who was first seen at the hospital six years previously with 'a breakdown'. This followed shortly upon him ending his relationship with his previous girlfriend, who was killed in a car accident one week later. A week after the accident, he was admitted to hospital with mutism and complaints that he kept seeing her face and hearing her voice. He was diagnosed as schizophrenic and started on regular haloperidol, but after spending three weeks in hospital he recovered fully and has remained well since. He has been off all medication for five years. The couple are now asking for advice about the risk that any children they have might subsequently develop schizophrenia.

Questions

1. What further information would you require and why?
2. Give rough estimates of developing schizophrenia in children, siblings, parents, and second degree relatives of patients with schizophrenia.
3. How would you present this information to the couple?
4. What is your estimate of the chances that the husband may suffer further such 'breakdowns'?

Answers

1. The couple are understandably concerned that the husband may be carrying a genetic predisposition to schizophrenia which he might pass on to their children. In order to clarify this, it would first be necessary to review the diagnosis for the husband's previous admission by obtaining his hospital notes. A three-week episode of mutism and hallucinations following major life events, and resolving fully, would not meet DSM-III-R criteria for schizophrenia, and it may well be that a more appropriate diagnosis is brief reactive psychosis, particularly in view of the good long-term outcome. It would also be important to establish the family histories of both the husband and the wife to see whether there were any cases of schizophrenia or other major mental illness in either pedigree. Finally, before giving any advice about the risks involved, it might be worthwhile asking them to consider what level of risk they would view as acceptable, and,

if they felt that the risks were unacceptable, what alternatives they propose, including having no children at all, or trying to adopt.

2. The lifetime risk of schizophrenia developing in somebody with no family history is approximately 1%. The lifetime risk in someone with a family history limited to second degree relatives, such as aunts or cousins, is approximately 2%–3%. Estimates of risks for closer relationships include: the parent of a schizophrenic 5%, a sibling 10%, mono-zygotic twin of a schizophrenic 50%–60%, the child of one schizophrenic parent 5%–15%, and a child of two schizophrenic parents 40%–50%. The risk appears to be increased if the schizophrenia in the proband is more severe in terms of early age of onset, chronicity, and lack of treatment response.

3. In view of the doubt about the husband's diagnosis, and his good subsequent outcome, and assuming that there is no other family history of schizophrenia, it might be best to frame the advice in the following terms: 'If there was no suggestion of schizophrenia in either of your families or yourselves, the risk that any child that you might have who would subsequently develop the condition is in the order of 1 in a 100. If the breakdown you suffered was a definite case of schizophrenia and had not turned out as well as it has, the risk that any children that you might have would develop the condition in later years would be of the order of 5%–15%, that is, 1 in 20 to 1 in 8 or so. However, since you recovered quickly and things have gone well subsequently, and since there is this uncertainly about the exact diagnosis involved, the risk to your children must be to the lower end of this range, at about 5%, or about 1 in 20. Your children are therefore at increased risk of developing schizophrenia, but the risk is still a relatively low one and it would not necessarily manifest itself for many years. You should take some time to consider this before coming to any decisions about whether to go ahead and have a family or not'.

4. The husband is employed, married and presumably in good physical health. If his diagnosis was definitely schizophrenia, all these would be pointers towards a relatively good long-term outcome, especially given the history of six years

without further relapse. If the diagnosis is of brief reactive psychosis, then, while he may expect similar symptoms after any subsequent major life events, the long-term prognosis for freedom from relapse is even better.

Case 7.1

A 13-year-old boy who has stopped attending school is brought for assessment. According to his mother, since he moved to a new school he has become withdrawn, and as the time of school approaches he becomes sweaty, complains of diarrhoea, starts to breathe heavily and absolutely refuses to go to school. On two occasions within the last month, when his father, who is usually abroad, put him in the car and took him to school, he managed to stay there all day.

Questions

1. How would you assess the situation?
2. What factors do you need to know to confirm the diagnosis?
3. What is his long-term prognosis?
4. How would you manage him?

Answers

1. The parents and the child should be seen together and separately to assess the history of the present difficulties. The parents should be asked for a full description of the current problem and associated emotional or intellectual difficulties. The functioning of the family is assessed with particular reference to the child's position in the family, by asking about the emotional environment at home, the physical and psychiatric health of family members, and the nature of the child's relationship with family members. A full developmental history of the child is taken, including his milestones and first reactions to kindergarten and/or school. Academic and social adjustments in school need to be assessed, so, with permission from the parents, school reports are obtained and contact established with the tutor. It is possible however that none of this information would identify the true cause of refusal in this case, so it would be important to see the child alone in a careful attempt to elicit fears (such as of bullying) that he has not so far dared to express.

2. The most obvious diagnosis appears to be school refusal. This usually stems from anxiety, especially in younger children, but older children may display a true phobic fear of aspects of school life. The usual pattern is of increasing

Case 7.1 decision tree

13-year-old boy not attending school

Kept at home by parents due to:
  work
  parental illness
  parental psychological problems

Involve school inspectors and legal authorities if necessary

Truancy
  parents unaware of absence
  poor achievers at school
  child does something he finds more interesting
  forerunner of delinquency

Involve family and social services

School refusal
  parents aware of absence
  high achievers
  child fearful of school or separation from parent
  forerunner of neurosis (when severe)

Treat associated depression. Behavioural approach, to return to school reluctance to go to school, which gradually leads to complete refusal. Such children may be overprotected and overdependent. Mothers may have neurotic difficulties of their own which may contribute to an ambivalent attitude to the child's school refusal. The fact that the child's father can get the child to attend while the mother cannot, suggests maternal ambivalence is relevant in this case. Somatic symptoms are common, as here. In earlier age groups it is common amongst girls, but around puberty boys tend to outnumber girls. In the latter age group, particularly, additional symptoms of depression may be seen, as suggested in this case.

3. Most younger children do return eventually but about one third of children with school refusal fail to return. Most of these are adolescents close to the school leaving age; they may do better at vocational training. An early diagnosis and early intervention with family co-operation improve the prognosis, but follow-up studies suggest a high rate of adult neurosis and social disability.

4. In the management, the most important factor is for the child to return to school. School teachers can be informed about the problem, and regular communication is of paramount importance. The child should be given a date to return to school, without any redress, after which he has to go every day. He should not be transferred to another school. Education welfare officers may be helpful in escorting the child to school regularly, if his mother finds this too difficult. Associated depression may need treatment in its own right.

Reference

Hersov, L. and Berg, I. (1980) *Out of School*. Wiley, Chichester

Case 7.2

A 78-year-old widower is assessed in casualty. He lives alone but is visited regularly by his nephew, who is his nearest relative. The nephew reports that when he visited recently, he found the patient to be very edgy and, when pressed, the patient said that he had been ' . . . seeing things' for the last few weeks. He reported seeing long-dead friends in his front room and becoming angry when they would not talk to him. He also described seeing small animals running around his kitchen. On being brought to hospital, he had become very agitated and had hit out at his nephew and nursing staff.

He retired as a builder, 10 years previously, on developing a cataract in his right eye. Corrective surgery had been unhelpful, and four years ago he developed a cataract in his left eye, but has refused treatment because he is terrified he will lose his sight completely.

On examination, he was cognitively intact and displayed no other psychiatric symptoms. The patient and his nephew confirm the absence of any previous psychiatric contact.

Questions

1. What would you do next?
2. If he refuses admission would you use the Mental Health Act?
3. Outline your assessment and management plan.
4. What do you know about Charles Bonnet syndrome?

Answers

1. This man is presenting with visual hallucinations and secondary agitation in late life, with no previous psychiatric history. A number of diagnoses present themselves, and he needs a period of in-patient assessment to establish the diagnosis and initiate treatment. He should be approached with tact and empathy, making it clear that the distressing nature of his symptoms is perfectly understood, and the aim of admission is to find the cause and treat it. It will be important to enlist the help of his nephew in persuading him to accept admission.
2. If attempts at persuading him to accept admission fail, then the question of applying the Mental Health Act arises. The degree of his agitation, and his hitting out at other people,

suggests that he may represent a danger to himself and others, and that the use of the Act is applicable. Furthermore, visual symptoms and agitation arising anew in elderly people, suggest the possibility of a delirium caused by serious but undetected underlying physical illness. Allowing him to leave hospital poses the risk that both the delirium and the underlying illness would deteriorate, threatening his health and possibly his life. It is probably best on balance to detain him.

3. Once admitted, the assessment would include taking a full psychiatric history from the patient, confirmed by an informant account from the nephew. A thorough Mental State Examination should be conducted, assessing particularly the presenting hallucinations and cognitive function. Nursing observation to detect any fluctuation in symptoms or level of consciousness and especially any nocturnal deterioration will be important. Physical examination will be needed to seek a possible underlying physical illness, and will need to be supplemented by baseline investigations with full blood count, erythrocyte sedimentation rate, biochemical screen, VDRL, thyroid function tests, B_{12} and folate, chest X-ray and a mid-stream urine (MSU). Depending on the results and his clinical progress, it may be appropriate to do a CT scan of the brain, an EEG, a lumbar puncture and blood cultures.

While this investigation is continuing, his general practitioner should be contacted for any information about any recent change of medication. It may be necessary to treat his agitation with sedating drugs and, in the elderly, low doses of neuroleptics, such as trifluoperazine, are preferable to benzodiazepines. He should be nursed in a brightly lit, quiet room, preferably by one or two nurses who can get to know him well, and with frequent visits from his nephew and other familiar people. As soon as his symptoms have subsided sufficiently, he should return home, initially for brief periods and then for longer periods, before being discharged. He will need out-patient supervision and may benefit from attending a day-centre.

4. Visual hallucinations in the elderly are normally accompanied by other features sufficient to diagnose an acute or sub-acute delirium, a dementing illness, or paraphrenia. The term 'Charles Bonnet syndrome' is reserved for the occurrence of persistent visual pseudohallucinations occurring in a state of clear consciousness, with preservation of insight. They are often very bizarre and vivid, and are usually associated with optical pathology. Various aetiologies have been suggested including undetected organic lesions, irritation of the visual cerebral cortex, and the result of visual sensory deprivation. The symptoms are usually resistant to treatment, and anti-psychotics appear to have little value. Anticonvulsants, such as carbamazepine, may be of benefit, but in most cases symptoms continue for prolonged periods without remission.

Case 7.2 decision tree

78-year-old man with visual hallucinations and agitation

Admit for assessment—under Section if necessary

Acute or sub-acute delirium

Identify cause via investigation and treat accordingly

Charles Bonnet syndrome
explain to patient
and family
try anticonvulsants
long-term support

Dementing illness

Exclude treatable cause.
Supportive treatment

Paraphrenia

Neuroleptic drugs.
Psychosocial support

Reference

Damas-Mora, J. et al. (1982) The Charles Bonnet syndrome in perspective. *Psychological Medicine*, **12** 251–261

Case 7.3

A 20-year-old male art student presents with a history of increasing withdrawal. He has been seen on two occasions by psychiatrists within the last year, and was noted to show 'obsessional slowness', but no further information is available. At interview, he complains that he has problems with examinations '. . . because my brain gets sticky.' As a child he was quiet, had few friends, and had problems separating from his parents at times of school camping trips etc. He did well at 'O' level and was expected to do well at 'A' level, but failed all his examinations. His parents were supportive and arranged for him to go to a private art school, which he has attended for eight months, saying that he enjoys it. He explains his withdrawal as a result of a loss of energy, due to him falling in love with his male art teacher. On examination, he is unkempt, unshaven, often vague in his responses, and frequently giggly and distractible. He denies any abnormal beliefs or experiences.

Questions

1. What differential diagnosis would you consider?
2. What further information or investigations would you like to confirm your diagnosis?
3. What would you tell his parents when they ask what is wrong with him?
4. How would you manage him if he accepts voluntary admission, but subsequently decides to leave the ward?

Answers

1. The patient presents with a gradual fall-off in academic performance, social withdrawal, poor self-care and suggestions of psychotic experiences. The most likely diagnosis is a first episode of schizophrenic illness, but alternatives include a major depressive episode, and drug-induced mental state changes.

2. The urine drug screen might confirm recent drug use, although it will not exclude such use nor will it confirm, if positive, that drug use is causally linked to the presenting symptoms. Other investigations might exclude rare organic causes of his presentation, but are unlikely to confirm or refute the diagnoses of schizophrenia or depressive psychosis. It will be more important to obtain an exhaustive history from his parents, his art school colleagues and tutors, his previous psychiatrists, his general practitioner and his school. If this information fails to reveal evidence of mood changes, or characteristic sleep and appetite disturbance of depression, then the diagnosis of schizophrenia becomes more likely. Detailed enquiries into his family history may reveal other cases with a similar diagnosis.

3. While the diagnosis remains uncertain, it is best not to use any diagnostic labels, such as schizophrenia, in discussion with his parents. With his consent, his parents should be told that he has a serious mental illness, whose character has not yet been determined, but which should become clearer with the passage of time. They should be told that his symptoms can be controlled with medication, and that with appropriate out-patient support he may well be able to return to his art school, or some alternative activity. The role of high levels of Expressed Emotion in precipitating relapse should be explained to them, and they should be told that his diagnosis will be kept under review after discharge, on the basis of his subsequent progress.

4. Many voluntary patients who wish to leave an in-patient unit do so impulsively, but can be dissuaded if their reasons for wishing to go can be elicited and attended to. If he is responding to high levels of disturbance on the ward and simply wishes to get away for a while, he could be offered

time off the ward in the company of a staff member. If he will not accept this, and remains unamenable to persuasion to stay, then the use of a Section 5 (2) in England and Wales (72 hour) holding order should be considered. In order to apply this, there would need to be evidence that he poses a risk to his own health or safety, or that he should be detained for the protection of other persons. At the same time that it is applied, consideration should be given to the use of a Section 2, although in many cases once the Section 5 (2) expires, patients are content to remain voluntarily.

Case 7.4

A 48-year-old man who in the past has had at least three courses of detoxification for his alcohol problems is referred for psychiatric assessment. He had approached his general practitioner, saying that he has morning shakes, and usually has his first drink at 8 am—as soon as he gets up. A publican by profession, his marriage broke up six months ago because of his inability to maintain erections.

Questions

1. How would you assess the problem?
2. What would you do for short-term management?
3. What do you know of the use of disulfiram?
4. What role do you think psychotherapy plays in the management of alcoholism?

Answers

1. This man appears to be a chronic alcoholic re-presenting for an attempt at treatment after previous failures. Assessment needs to take into account the biological, psychological and social aspects of his drinking and its consequences. To assess the former, his drinking habits need to be quantified,

and his past medical history and any current physical symptoms reviewed, as well as undertaking a physical examination and investigation (including a blood count, liver function tests, and serum B_{12} and folate). Assessment of psychological aspects requires a full psychiatric history and mental state examination, if he is sober enough to co-operate. Associated psychological disorders, particularly anxiety and depression, need to be identified if they are present, as do the various direct psychological manifestations of alcoholism, including intoxication, withdrawal anxiety and early delirium tremens, and alcoholic hallucinosis. His current motivation to change his pattern of drinking also needs to be established. Finally, the effects of his drinking upon his job, and his social relationships, need to be reviewed.

Perhaps the most important questions to consider are why he is re-presenting now, and why previous treatments failed.

2. His immediate management depends on his presentation and the help he is seeking. If he is intoxicated, he should be told to return later when sober. If he is seeking help to stop drinking, then detoxification is indicated. This may need to be undertaken as an in-patient, facilities permitting, if his previous detoxification failures were as an out-patient. He will need regular observation, rehydration and nutrition, vitamin supplementation with vitamin B compound, and a reducing course of chlordiazepoxide over 7–10 days. If there is evidence of delirium tremens developing he needs admission to a medical ward for the above measures together with rehydration (parenterally if necessary) and treatment of any underlying physical illness.

Once he is detoxified and alcohol-free, attention can be directed at the various longer-term management options available to keep him abstinent, including referral to Alcoholics Anonymous, or residential rehabilitation units, or continuing out-patient care.

3. Disulfiram, or Antabuse, acts by inhibiting a liver enzyme involved in the metabolism of alcohol, acetaldehyde dehydrogenase. If a patient on disulfiram drinks alcohol, the blood levels of acetaldehyde rise, causing within minutes an unpleasant syndrome of flushing, headache, palpitations,

tachycardia, nausea and vomiting. It therefore may help to reduce drinking through behavioural mechanisms (a conditioning process, where the unpleasant symptoms are associated with alcohol) and cognitive factors (patients know they will experience the reaction and therefore find ways to avoid drinking).

There are risks attached; for some patients the reactions are severe, with hypotensive collapse requiring emergency treatment. Even the small amounts of alcohol in cough medicine may be enough to trigger a reaction; reactions have been reported following the use of shampoos containing alcohol; patients should be forewarned and should carry a treatment card. Disulfiram should be avoided in cardiac disease, epilepsy, pregnancy or psychosis, and can cause side-effects of fatigue, nausea, and psychotic episodes. It also interferes with the hepatic metabolism of other drugs, notably warfarin.

It is given as an initial single dose of 800 mg, having warned the patient to avoid alcohol for 12 hours beforehand. The dose is then reduced over five days to 100–200 mg daily. Enzyme inhibition continues for about four days after the last dose, so alcohol reactions can still occur in this period.

4. An overview of the evidence suggests that there are no striking differences in outcome between the various forms of psychological treatments of alcoholism, and that factors within the patient are more important than the details of the treatment offered. For this reason, it is hard to justify long-term or intensive individual treatment. Group treatment is widely used, and although most of it is conducted in out-patient clinics, there is a place for in-patient or residential group rehabilitation units, as well as the informal group sessions offered by Alcoholics Anonymous. Recently, research has begun to consider treatment along behavioural lines, using graded exposure to cues for drinking with response prevention. Initial results are encouraging but it is too soon for this treatment to be generally recommended (Rankin, 1983). For some patients, who find groups too threatening, the best approach is a supportive one, using problem-solving methods.

Whatever approach is adopted, there is still controversy whether the aim should be complete abstinence or controlled drinking.

Reference

Rankin, H. et al. (1983) Cue exposure and response prevention with alcoholism: a controlled trial. *Behavioural Research and Therapy*, **21**, 435–46

Case 8.1

A 27-year-old woman presents complaining of sudden feelings of anxiety associated with palpitations, vertigo and a fear of fainting. These have been going on for some months, and now occur almost weekly, lasting several minutes at a time. The general practitioner's referral letter mentions that the patient's mother is described as paranoid, and that her paternal grandfather had schizophrenia. She is unmarried, and isolated from her family who live abroad.

Questions

1. What else would you like to know from her and about her in order to reach a diagnosis?
2. What, in your view, is the most likely diagnosis, and what prognostic implications does it have?
3. What range of treatments is available for this patient?
4. What approach might a cognitive therapist take to such a case?

Answers

1. Compilation of the history should attend to three areas, including, firstly, further details of the presenting symptoms and their associated features. For example, does the anxiety come on without warning, or is it associated with particular circumstances? Are there associated features of anxiety, such as sweating, tremor, or disturbance of bowel or bladder functioning? Has she ever actually fainted? Does she avoid certain activities or circumstances which she fears might set off an attack? The second area of enquiry should cover any symptoms *between* episodes, examining whether there is any evidence of depression or anxiety and whether she is functioning normally in other respects. Thirdly, her personal history needs to be fully considered, particularly regarding her premorbid functioning and any recent life events. Although her family live abroad, it would be

valuable to get information from an informant who has witnessed an attack and who could describe any overall changes in the patient since the attacks began.

2. The patient is describing panic attacks and the most likely diagnosis is panic disorder. This is commonly associated with agoraphobic avoidance of precipitating circumstances. Panic attacks may arise in the context of another disorder; and, occasionally, they may be the result of organic dysfunction, particularly that of the thyroid system. Although there is nothing in the current history to suggest it, her family history raises the question of schizophrenia. It is possible that she is experiencing auditory hallucinations which she is reluctant to describe, and that her anxiety attacks are entirely secondary to this.

   Where panic attacks are secondary to an underlying disorder, most commonly depression, prognosis will parallel that of the underlying disorder. Less is known about the long-term prognosis of panic disorder *per se*, but it is not uncommon for distressing and disabling symptoms to persist for years before treatment is sought. In such circumstances, treatment is usually difficult.

3. The range of treatments suggested for panic disorder indicates the range of aetiological explanations offered. For some patients, a tendency to acute or chronic hyperventilation is the primary dysfunction, and panic attacks are secondary to the effects of hypocapnia. In such cases, breathing exercises, together with demonstration of the effects of over-breathing during hyperventilation provocation tests, can be of great value. An alternative aetiological explanation stresses the biochemical abnormalities of panic disorder, and provides the justification for drug treatment. Tricyclic antidepressants, particularly imipramine, and less frequently MAOIs, particularly phenelzine, have been used to good effect. Benzodiazepines carry the risk of dependence, and are less useful, and, although a role for alprazolam has been claimed, this remains controversial. For all drug treatments, there is a significant risk of relapse upon withdrawal of drug treatment. This is particularly worrying in the case of benzodiazepines. A third aetiological explanation stresses cognitive misinterpretation as a central pathology

and suggests that panic attacks arise from a vicious circle where excessive awareness of bodily sensations generates anxiety about illness, which in turn has physical manifestations, which are themselves a cause of further anxiety.

4. The aim of cognitive therapy is to train the patient to identify and challenge inappropriate cognitive interpretations of

Case 8.1 decision tree

27-year-old woman. Episodic anxiety

Detailed assessment
  nature of the episode
  condition between episodes
  personal history
  medication use

Underlying depression or other psychiatric disorder

Treat accordingly

Underlying physical abnormality (e.g. thyroid disease) or use of anxiogenic substance (e.g. caffeinism)

Treat accordingly

Panic disorder

Drugs
  imipramine
  phenelzine
  alprazolam

Cognitive behaviour therapy

physical sensations so as to break the vicious circle referred to above. At a detailed initial assessment, much attention will be paid to the thoughts going through the patient's mind before and during the panic attack. For example, patients may fear that palpitations imply an impending heart attack and therefore may become extremely anxious every time their heart rate rises. Such fears can be identified and challenged during treatment sessions, and by use of diaries and homework between sessions, in such a way that the patients can learn to challenge the fears themselves. A substantial benefit of cognitive therapy arises from the persistence of its effects after a course of treatment has ended, in contrast to drug treatment.

Reference

Clark, D.M. (1986) A cognitive approach to panic. *Behaviour Research and Therapy*, **24**, 461–470

Case 8.2

An 11-year-old girl of Jamaican origin who was brought up by her grandparents is brought for assessment. She joined her parents in the UK 18 months ago and since her arrival she has been getting into scrapes both at school and at home. She hates the country and the weather and finds it difficult to relate to her parents. On interview, she says that they 'expect me to be their slave'. In addition to her school work she is expected to do the housework because both her parents are at work. She has no history of any problems prior to her arrival and she said that she had been very happy and contented. On examination, you find her low in spirits and she expresses feelings of wanting to run away from her parents back to her grandmother. She hates all the name calling she experiences and finds it difficult to make any friends.

Questions

1. What is your opinion about this case?
2. What will you communicate to her parents?
3. How will you manage her?
4. What do you understand of the relationship between migration and psychiatric disorder?

Answers

1. It would appear that this girl is expressing her anger and frustration at being moved to another culture and finding it difficult to accept her parents and their expectations. There is no evidence that she suffers from any major psychiatric disorder. It would appear that she has an adjustment reaction with a depressive element. Her problems may have been compounded by her parents' expectations of her.

2. The parents need to be reassured that the condition is transient and should subside without any specific intervention. However, they must be sensitive to her needs and acknowledge the difficulties that she has to get over in making new friends and settling down. She may need to grieve for her separation from her grandparents and then be encouraged to develop independence.

3. She should be seen for a fixed number of sessions initially by herself and then with the family to convey and work through her feelings of anger, frustration and loss. No medication is required. Liaison with her school's welfare officer and with social services will be important.

4. Much research has compared the rates of psychiatric disorder among immigrants with that among the indigenous population, and there is a consensus that many immigrant groups are at increased risk of many psychiatric conditions, though this is not universal. Some groups appear to be at *reduced* risk for some conditions. There are many competing explanations for the relative risks revealed, at social, cultural and biological levels. For example, the increased risk of schizophrenia among first-(and especially second-) generation Afro-Caribbean immigrants to the UK has been

claimed to be caused by selective migration of vulnerable individuals, the social disadvantage and racist rejection these immigrants meet with, and the exposure of immunologically vulnerable pregnant women to unfamiliar viruses which affect brain development *in utero*. It is likely to be some time before these various explanations can be teased apart.

Case 8.3

A 29-year-old woman is charged with drowning her 4-year-old son in the bathtub. When she was seen in the out-patient clinic on two previous occasions, there was no evidence of mental illness, and her medical care is not seen as negligent. She had separated from her husband who had taken the other two children with him. Her solicitors require a psychiatric opinion to be presented by an expert witness to the court on their behalf.

Questions

1. How would you proceed?
2. How would you decide fitness to plead?
3. What would your recommendations to the courts be?

Answers

1. The legal representative's request would need to be clarified in writing and all appropriate information should be sought including prosecution statements, indictments, proof of evidence, other medical and social reports, and a review of her case notes. The accused should be seen and after explaining the altered confidentiality of the interview, her history and mental state should be assessed. The aim should be to formulate an understanding as to why the offence was committed. How the patient is pleading should be taken into account in order to assess the implications of her answers.

Her fitness to plead needs to be assessed, as does her responsibility at the time of the offence, the presence of mental disorder, the possible disposal options, and her prognosis, as well as an explanation of the offence. The legal representatives should be advised accordingly, making recommendations for management.

2. To be fit to plead at the time of a trial, a defendant must be able to understand the charge and his/her plea to it, to challenge a juror, to instruct counsel, to examine a witness, and to follow the progress of the trial. The issue of fitness to plead can be raised by defence, prosecution or judge, often on the basis of medical reports; but the decision is always made by a jury. If found unfit to plead, the defendant is committed to a special hospital as directed by the Home Secretary, until such time as he discharges them or they later become fit to plead.

3. Recommendations cannot be made without having conducted a full assessment, as outlined. On the basis of that assessment, the aim in making recommendations would be to help the court come to an understanding of the offence and the importance of any underlying mental disorder or mitigating factors; to give an estimate of the defendant's prognosis and future dangerousness, and to offer or to recommend whatever disposal and treatment might be most appropriate.

Case 8.4

A request is made for an assessment of a 23-year-old male student in a hall of residence in the local university. The university health service doctor is present, and says that the student's long-term homosexual partner had left him recently because of repeated groundless accusations of infidelity. Two days ago the student had seen his doctor complaining that the academic staff were conspiring to prevent him from getting a degree: the doctor had given him a week's supply of amitriptyline. Now the student has locked himself in and refuses to 'face the world'.

Questions

1. What would you do?
2. What kind of mood changes can you expect?
3. How would you deal with him in the long-term management?

Answers

1. Before trying to talk with him, it would be important to gather as much information as possible in the time available. His doctor should be asked about his past mental and psychiatric history and his mental state when seen most recently, and his friends and tutor should be asked about his personality and academic record, any recent changes in him, and any evidence of drug abuse.

   Armed with this information, a friend he trusts should be asked to introduce him, and then he should be talked to through the door. This approach would need to be patient and tactful, and care should be taken not to appear threatening. The aim should be to persuade him to open the door so as to speak more freely with him. An appeal to confidentiality might help: as he is paranoid, he may well worry about conversations regarding his personal life and feelings being shouted through a door for all to hear.

   If he agrees to be seen, as full an assessment as possible should then be conducted. It is important to ensure one's own safety and the safety of those nearby: paranoid patients may become violent if they feel particularly threatened, and he may well view a psychiatrist as an agent of the university authorities. If he does not agree to be seen, and there is sufficient evidence to indicate a high risk to himself or to others, then it is advisable to consider involving the university security service and the police in making a forced entry. If there is no such risk, the best policy might be to leave him alone for a 'cooling off period', perhaps with friends nearby, while arranging to call again the following day.

2. Persecutory beliefs and preoccupations can arise with other symptoms in a number of different psychiatric disorders, or alternatively may be the only presenting symptom. They

can therefore be associated with widely differing mood states. If they arise in a manic episode they may be associated with expansive grandiosity and boastful egocentricity; if in a depressive episode, with low mood, self-criticism and guilt. Persecutory beliefs arising in schizophrenia may be accompanied by a flattened affect without the extremes seen in manic depressive illness.

3. His management depends on his diagnosis, which must first be established through a period of assessment, preferably as an in-patient, under a section of the Mental Health Act if necessary.

There is probably sufficient evidence of a serious mental disorder to justify this, although arriving at a precise diagnosis will take more time. Depending on the diagnosis, his future management will involve pharmacological and psychosocial aspects of treatment. He is likely to require neuroleptic medication, such as haloperidol, together with drugs for any underlying mood disorder. Close liaison will be required with the student health doctor and the academic staff. If he leaves university (or is asked to), it will be important that his general practitioner and the psychiatric services in his home town are informed about his condition and its treatment. Of particular concern in this case is his homosexuality, which raises the issue of human immunodeficiency virus (HIV) related CNS disease as a diagnostic possibility; and, more importantly, which will require careful attention to confidentiality in dealing with other services and his family, who may not know and whom he may wish not to be informed.

Especially where the symptoms arise in isolation, as part of one of the paranoid disorders (including, as in this case, morbid jealousy), they may well be associated with considerable anger and hostility directed towards their presumed persecutors. If this is so, there is a significant risk of violence, and an assessment of dangerousness is mandatory.

Patients with persecutory beliefs are likely to see any interviewers as potential further persecutors. They are therefore commonly distant, reserved and unforthcoming, especially in the early stages of interview.

Case 9.1

A 68-year-old retired accountant, who describes himself as a life-long perfectionist, presents with a two-year history of 'being infested with fleas'. He has been to see various dermatologists privately but without any improvement. He now feels angry that no one takes him seriously, and he is particularly frustrated at being referred to a psychiatrist. He retired three years previously and, according to his wife, during the first year of his retirement he would drink up to three bottles of wine a day to overcome his boredom. He stopped drinking altogether after a severe attack of angina, and is now not on any medication. On examination, his sensorium and cognitive functions are normal, as is his mood, although he has a marked fine tremor of both hands. His conviction about being infested with fleas is unshakeable, although he shows no other abnormal beliefs or experiences.

Questions

1. What is your differential diagnosis?
2. You begin treatment with pimozide, 4 mg at night, but on follow-up, three weeks later, you discover that his beliefs about the fleas are still unshakeable, and he has only been taking the medication on alternate days. How would you improve his compliance?
3. What is his long-term prognosis?

Answers

1. The patient displays a delusional belief of infestation. Delusional parasitosis of this type occasionally arises in schizophrenia, psychotic depression, or organically based psychotic illnesses, but there is no evidence from the rest of the history to suggest any of these as the appropriate diagnosis. It is therefore most likely that he has a mono-symptomatic hypochondriacal psychosis, which would be classified

under paranoia in the ICD-9 system, or with delusional disorder, somatic type, in the DSM-III-R system. These conditions are relatively rare, generally begin in middle age or late life, and are associated with socially isolating changes, such as immigration or deafness (Munro, 1988). The delusion is usually well encapsulated, so that the level of function is good overall. Secondary depression is common, and a history of alcohol or drug abuse seem to be over-represented compared with the normal population. Claims have been made for a variety of treatment agents, but the best evidence in support of benefits applies to the anti-psychotic pimozide.

2. Compliance is a major problem in this group. They generally resent referrals to psychiatrists, believing with unshakeable conviction that their problem is dermatological rather than psychiatric.

The best way to try to improve this man's compliance might be to enter into an informal contract with him. He might be told that in order to assess whether pimozide is of any benefit he needs an adequate treatment trial for a specified period, for example, one month. He could therefore be asked to take the pimozide as prescribed for this period, whatever his views about its effects, and then at the end of one month to discuss with the psychiatrist his view about the outcome. If his poor compliance is partly due to troublesome side-effects, these might be minimized by changing the time of day at which he takes the drug, and by prescription of an anti-cholinergic agent at the same time. If it is a matter of forgetting to take the medication, then his wife might be recruited to remind him, or simple behavioural strategies might be employed, such as always taking the drug immediately after cleaning his teeth at night.

Another way of improving compliance might be to focus on non-drug methods of treatment in addition. Social isolation commonly accompanies retirement, and may be a causal factor in this case. He might be encouraged to take up part-time work, or put in touch with local clubs for the retired, day-centres, or voluntary agencies. Again, his wife could be enlisted in attempting to interest him in alternative activities.

3. Left untreated, these disorders may continue unchanged for many years. Therefore, if he persists in non-compliance, his course is likely to be a chronic one. He may benefit from pimozide, but is likely to require maintenance treatment for the rest of his life. Conversely, there is little evidence of generalization of psychotic symptoms to other areas of life, or of an overall deterioration in level of functioning with the passage of time.

Reference

Munro, A. (1988) Mono-symptomatic hypochondriacal psychosis. *British Journal of Psychiatry*, **153**, 37–40

Case 9.2

The duty social worker has requested an assessment of a 5-year-old girl as a matter of urgency. The social worker had gone to see the mother at the request of the general practitioner. The mother had been feeling depressed and the social worker felt that the child was 'manic'. The mother had a manic episode several years ago. The child had been running around the flat and was noted to be very distractible.

Questions

1. What would you like to achieve in interviewing the parents? Give your differential diagnosis.
2. What are the early predictors of hyperactivity?
3. Outline your management plans.
4. Can you tell us something about the mode of functioning of methyl phenidate?

Answers

1. The parental interview is an indispensable part of the assessment of children with behavioural problems. First, such an interview enables a rapport to be established with the parents and the child and a description of the parental view of the child's problem to be obtained, which would in turn enable the focus to be narrowed for direct observations. Secondly, the child may be more amenable to interview having seen her parents in the same situation. The parental interview will also involve parents in the diagnostic process and treatment programme.

    The most likely diagnosis in this case is hyperactivity or hyperkinetic syndrome. This is characterized by persistent, purposeless motor activity, a limited attention span, distractibility, impulsivity and emotional instability. It may be associated with CNS maturational delay and mental handicap or autism. Although it is highly unlikely in this age group, in view of the family history a manic episode needs to be excluded.

2. A history of hyperactivity in one or both parents or alcoholism and sociopathy have been reported to be associated with hyperactivity. Soft neurological signs and EEG abnormalities have been linked to the condition, particularly in American samples, and abnormalities of infant temperament (comprising habit regularity, reactivity to stimulation, activity level, irritability, withdrawal and negative mood) may also be linked.

3. None of these associations is very clear, but the first step is to assess whether the descriptions are justified and the diagnosis of hyperactivity applies. If the behaviour is regarded as abnormal, parental education and the establishment of a behavioural programme is the first line of treatment. Remedial education and family therapy may be indicated. Drugs may have an important role to play. Methylphenidate 5–20 mg/day may be used though this can be increased up to 80 mg/day. Dextroamphetamine can be used but should be given earlier in the day, since it is likely to keep the child awake. Phenothiazines and haloperidol can be used as well.

4. Stimulants, such as methylphenidate and dextroamphetamine, are used in hyperactive children on the hypothesis
   that affected children have under-active reticular activating
   systems and hence insufficient cortical inhibitory control,
   and the fact that the ᴄ ⁻ᵍgs are effective provides evidence to
   support this hypothesis. Both drugs improve concentration,
   reduce impulsivity and make purposeless activity more goal
   directed. There are various side-effects, including growth
   retardation, insomnia and depression.

Case 9.3

A 26-year-old secretary has been referred for psychiatric
assessment by her general practitioner. She notes that the
patient suffers from severe anxiety symptoms when she thinks
of spiders. The problem has been present for most of her life.
The patient and her husband are going on a safari holiday in six
week's time and she is absolutely petrified that she will be
faced with a spider and die. There is no other psychiatric problem.

Questions

1. How would you assess this patient?
2. How would you treat her?
3. What advice would you give to the husband?
4. What medication would you prescribe?

Answers

1. She appears to be suffering from an animal phobia—a relatively common, simple or monosymptomatic phobic disorder, more common in females and generally beginning in
   childhood.

   There are usually few other symptoms but, occasionally, a
   depressive illness can co-exist with the phobia. Assessment

should therefore include a sufficiently detailed psychiatric history and mental state examination to exclude depression and other conditions, and to establish the extent of self-medication with alcohol or other drugs. A detailed behavioural description of the symptoms should be taken. This should cover their onset, intensity and duration, and the extent of any anticipatory anxiety or avoidance, as well as a hierarchy of feared situations involving spiders, and the clarification of definite treatment goals. The patient's motivation to engage in treatment, and the willingness of her husband to act as co-therapist should also be assessed.

2. The treatment of choice is behavioural psychotherapy. The rationale behind the treatment, and its co-operative nature, should first be clearly explained to the patient, who should then be taught simple relaxation techniques such as progressive muscular relaxation. The patient will then be exposed to a graded series of feared situations, and will be encouraged to remain in each situation until her anxiety subsides. She will be asked to record her anxiety levels before, during and after treatment, on a simple chart. Exposure *in vivo* is more effective than exposure in imagination, but if she finds even the lowest level of the former intolerable, treatment may need to begin with the latter, and progress later to *in vivo* work. A hierarchy of exposure should be constructed through discussion with her, which might begin with pictures of spiders, and progress through dead spiders in a covered box in the corner of the room, to a living spider in the patient's hand, via a series of stages. Between sessions, the patient should practice these exposures at home, with the help of her husband, and record the results for discussion at the next session.

3. The husband should be involved throughout as co-therapist. The principles underlying the treatment should be explained to him, so that he clearly understands what is expected of him. He should be encouraged to help maintain the patient's motivation for her homework sessions, and should be told that with his help, her efforts, and weekly sessions, her fear of spiders should be greatly reduced in the six weeks remaining before their holiday.

4. No medication should be prescribed. Anxiolytics, MAOIs and tricyclic antidepressants have all been used in phobic disorders. Although they may relieve distress in the short-term, there is a high relapse rate on stopping them, and, with the benzodiazapines, a risk of dependence. In this case, if behavioural methods cannot be offered until the patient returns from holiday, it may be worth trying a short course of imipramine to cover the time the patient is away, but overall it is best avoided.

Case 9.4

You have been asked by the courts to assess a 46-year-old widower who has been loitering near school playgrounds and on two occasions has indecently exposed himself to children. He has not attacked, or forced intercourse on, or even touched any children so far as is known.

Questions

1. What factors would you bear in mind when you are assessing him?
2. Suppose the court discharges him on probation, with treatment as a condition. What treatment can you offer him?
3. What is his prognosis likely to be?

Answers

1. This man appears to be an exhibitionist, who gains sexual gratification from exposing his genitals to others without attempting any further contact. To understand more clearly the nature of his disorder, enquiries need to cover the details of his offences and his mood before and after, as well as his sexual development, his personality, and his current mental state. Exhibitionism has been subdivided into two types which differ in their prognosis and their response to

criminal proceedings and treatment (Rooth, 1971). Type I exhibitionists are said to be immature and inhibited, to experience mounting tension before exposing themselves, and guilt afterwards. Type II is characterized by sociopathic personality traits, masturbation during exposure, and subsequently, sadistic pleasure rather than guilt. It is relatively unusual for exhibitionism to present in middle age, and where it does, it suggests underlying organic brain damage, alcoholism, or a depressive illness. This man therefore needs a careful history, mental state and physical examination to exclude these possibilities. A history of his sexual relationship with his late wife should help establish the aetiological importance of her death. If he had always had an unsatisfactory sex life with her, he may well have had exhibitionist fantasies, but only now has begun to act on them or to get caught.

Alternatively, if his sex life was a fulfilling one, it is possible that his current behaviour has arisen in the context of a depressive illness following his wife's death.

Assessment should also cover some estimate of his likely dangerousness to other witnesses of his exposure. The account of his offences suggests a low risk, but any evidence of masturbation during exposure, or attempts at verbal or physical contact with the victim, all indicate a greater risk of sexual aggression in the future.

2. Any underlying disorder first needs to be identified and treated in its own right. Most exhibitionists do not re-offend after a first conviction, and psychiatric treatment is therefore reserved for repeat offenders, as this man appears to be. Drug treatment with anti-androgen agents, such as cyproterone, has been used, but there are risks and side-effects, and the benefits are uncertain, so this course is not generally recommended. This would need informed consent. Psychoanalytic approaches for individuals and groups have also been adopted, but evidence about efficacy is lacking. Treatment along behavioural lines is therefore the preferred option. Aversive therapy with electrical shocks has been reported to help, but there are major ethical problems and the treatment has not become established. Covert sensitization is a technique in which the patient is asked to imagine,

rather than experience, adverse consequences (such as arrest, publicity, court appearances and so on) and to associate these with the act of exposure. When coupled with social skills training and relaxation techniques to reduce the pre-exposure anxiety, this may be the best treatment, but even then a substantial proportion of patients will continue to offend.

3. Type II exhibitionists, especially those who attempt physical contact with the victim or select particularly young victims, have a poor prognosis, as do those where the behaviour emerges as a result of brain damage. Type I exhibitionists with otherwise stable lives and supportive spouses do better, especially if well-motivated to engage in behavioural treatment.

This man does not clearly fit either category, and his prognosis is likely to be that of any underlying condition if his exhibitionism has only recently emerged.

The fact that he has repeated his offence already, is a poor prognostic indicator.

Case 10.1

At the end of an afternoon clinic, a 68-year-old woman presents who, according to the general practitioner's letter, is 'severely depressed'. She arrives accompanied by her 72-year-old husband, who says that she has eaten very little over the last five days and has on two occasions said that she wished she were dead. She appears dishevelled, shows marked psychomotor retardation and admits feeling hopeless, helpless and worthless. She is unable to see any future. Her illness started three weeks after her sister-in-law's sudden death. She was very close to the sister-in-law, but managed to cope with the funeral arrangements. It is late Friday afternoon, prior to a long Bank Holiday weekend. You suggest that she be admitted. She refuses.

Questions

1. Outline your plan of management.
2. After 24 hours in the ward, you find that she has completely stopped eating and drinking and she is becoming dehydrated. What would you do next?
3. In this case, how long would you recommend that she continues with her antidepressants?

Answers

1. It would appear from the history that she is severely depressed and needs admission. This option should be discussed with her husband and any other family member who may be able to persuade her to come in voluntarily. If they are unable to do so, but agree with the admission in principle, one of the Sections of the Mental Health Act can be used. If they disagree and are able to look after her at home and keep an eye on her, it might be necessary to discuss the options with the consultant and allow her to go home, with an option to bring her back into the hospital if her condition deteriorates. The general practitioner should be informed

and the plan discussed with him or her. If the family agree to a Section the duty social worker should be asked to apply for a Section 2 (in England or Wales). Any physical causes of her depression—in particular myxoedema and vitamin B_{12} or folate deficiencies should be ruled out. If at all possible,

Case 10.1 decision tree

she should be observed on the ward, initially without any medication, and her family history, personal history, premorbid personality and past history assessed, to arrive at a confident diagnosis before beginning treatment.

2. She requires close monitoring of fluid intake, rehydration, and correction of any electrolyte imbalance. If intensive nursing cannot persuade her to take fluid orally, she may need a nasogastric tube or intravenous infusion. She now requires treatment without delay for a presumptive diagnosis of depression and, accordingly, ECT is indicated, possibly on an emergency basis over the weekend. There is now good evidence that her mental state poses a risk to her health, which would warrant the application of a Section of the Mental Health Act, if she is still a voluntary patient and remains ambivalent about admission or reluctant to accept treatment. If she refuses ECT, this might need to be given following a second opinion from the Mental Health Act Commission (the Mental Welfare Commission in Scotland). She would need to be on a Section 2 or 3 for this, and if the administrative delays involved pose a risk to her health, one or two applications of ECT might first need to be given under Section 62 of the Mental Health Act (or Section 102 in Scotland).

3. Normally, it is recommended that after recovery the patient should continue on the medication for at least six months. The dosage of the antidepressants can be reduced to maintenance levels, (usually about half the effective treatment dose) and then gradually withdrawn.

If the patient tolerates treatment well, and the depressive episode was severe, as in this case, then it would be appropriate to continue for longer, especially if the patient shows evidence of periods of lowered mood while on maintenance treatment. Any depressive symptom emerging on withdrawal should be detected early and treated vigorously.

Case 10.2

An educational psychologist is concerned about an 8-year-old boy who has started shouting obscenities in class. These started to occur about 10 days ago and occur without any prov-ocation. On one occasion the teacher reported that he was putting it on because he had not done his homework. Prior to this, he had been an above average student.

Questions

1. What advice would you offer the educational psychologist?
2. What are the possible causes of this condition?
3. How would you manage this condition?
4. Give the short-term and long-term prognosis.

Answers

1. Habit spasms or tics, of which Gilles de la Tourette syndrome appears variant, is a fairly common condition. About 5% of 5–7-year old children give a history of tics. It is important to ascertain whether this child had motor tics as well as obscene utterances. The vocal tics may demonstrate echolalia. After gaining background information, the advice to the educational psychologist is to contact the parents and arrange an out-patient appointment. The motor tics often affect the face, and eye-blinking tics are one of the most common types.
2. The exact cause is not known though various hypotheses have been proposed. Among the proposed causes are included emotional tension, brain damage or developmental abnormality. Explanations from learning theory have been put forward. Some authors have reported reduced turnovers of serotonin and dopamine in the brain. The tics are more common in children, especially younger ones, and affect boys more commonly. Some authors have commented that these tics are means of expressing anxiety and aggression in individuals who may have difficulty in expressing these emotions more directly.
3. The general management includes support along with the removal or alleviation of any circumstances causing anxiety in the child. Parents and teachers should be encouraged to

ignore the tics and these could be explained as somatic manifestation of anxiety. In severe cases, as well as in Gilles de la Tourette syndrome, haloperidol, in small doses (up to 6 mg daily), or pimozide have been found useful. Psychotherapy is of the supportive variety. Behaviour therapy, especially satiation, has been shown to work in some cases.

4. If this is Gilles de la Tourette syndrome, haloperidol usually brings improvement. In long-term (four-year follow-up) 40% of children had recovered, though anxiety and neurotic symptoms have been reported in follow-ups.

Case 10.3

The local school headmaster is concerned that some of his 13–14-year-old students are beginning to abuse solvents. He has found a lot of empty canisters and aerosols lying around. He wants to know what symptoms he should be looking for.

Questions

1. What do you tell him?
2. How do you think you should manage those who have been abusing solvents and are referred to you?
3. What is the general prognosis in such cases?

Answers

1. Volatile solvents, such as glue, cleaning fluids, petrol and butane gas, are abused by about 10% of young people, usually by inhalation from a plastic bag. Inhalation produces euphoria, which can progress to disorientation, hallucinations, dysphasia and dysarthria and, finally, drowsiness and stupor, in a sequence similar to that of alcohol intoxication but arising and resolving much more quickly. Use is most common among boys aged 13–15 years, and tends to occur in groups on an occasional and experimental basis, without

long-term adverse effects. A small proportion go on to regular long-term use, with evidence of psychological but not
physical dependence, and adverse effects on health, including death due to accidents, cardiac arrhythmias and liver
toxicity.

Users will have the smell of the solvent on their breath and
on their clothes, and may show evidence of transient intoxication, disorientation and hallucinations. Chronic abusers
may have a characteristic peri-oral rash from repeated inhalation, and may show evidence of weight loss and broncho-
spasm. Solvent abusers predominantly tend to be boys,
from broken homes, who have poor academic records or
are unemployed. They come from all social classes, though
those with lower class backgrounds are over-represented.
They commonly also abuse alcohol and other drugs, and, if
abuse becomes chronic, they often acquire delinquent characteristics and criminal records.

2. Little is known about how to treat established solvent abuse,
and despite some reports of success with out-patient family
therapy, there is a general view that outcome is poor. The
emphasis is therefore on prevention, through educational
services based in schools and the community—though it has
been argued that increasing publicity will actually generate
more solvent abuse than it prevents.

As with all substance abuse disorders, the patient's motivation to change is a major determinant of outcome, but this
is harder to assess in adolescents than adults, especially
since peer pressure is such a strong force leading to abuse.
Working with adolescents and their families on underlying
problems pre-dating or perpetuating the abuse may well be
the best available approach for that small proportion who do
present to treatment services voluntarily. Others, who come
via the criminal justice system, pose different problems and
are likely to do badly whatever treatment is offered.

3. There is sparse information about outcome. Most children
who abuse solvents do so occasionally, for a short time, and
then either give up or move on to alcohol and other drugs.
Approximately 10% of occasional abusers go on to regular
solitary use. If they ever enter treatment, it will be through

the courts, and with poor motivation; both factors indicate a poor outcome.

There is nothing to indicate that the pupils the headmaster is concerned about are likely to fall into this category.

Case 10.4

A 37-year-old white man presented to the casualty department with complaints that he was being persecuted and could hear the voices of his persecutors plotting against him. He was unable to say anything about his family and friends, saying that he lived by himself. He admitted that he had not slept for several days because he was convinced that his persecutors would kill him if he slept. He said that he had had a similar episode ten years ago which lasted ten days. He has no other psychiatric history and said that he is still working as a hotel porter—a job that he has held for 12 years or so. There was no alcohol on his breath, and a physical examination was normal.

Questions

1. What is your differential diagnosis?
2. Outline your short-term management.
3. What is his prognosis?

Answers

1. This man is clearly psychotic, but the nature of his psychosis remains unclear. Paranoid schizophrenia is a possibility, but the short duration of the previous episode and evidence, from his continued employment, of good function between episodes mitigate against it. If there is evidence of psychosocial stress or major life events preceding both the current and previous episodes, then a diagnosis of brief reactive psychosis could be entertained. It is possible, for example, that he is someone whose fragile equilibrium has been

disturbed by changes in his role at work. A drug-induced psychosis is another possibility, and he will require a urine drug screen and a drug history to exclude it. Finally, there are rare organic causes of intermittent short-lived psychotic episodes, such as acute intermittent porphyria or endocrine abnormalities which need to be excluded.

2. He needs admission to a general psychiatric ward, for a few days of drug-free observation and intensive information-gathering, including obtaining the details of his previous episodes. This will allow a provisional diagnosis to be made; but whatever the diagnosis is, he is likely to need antipsychotic medication, at least in the short term. If he clearly responded to a particular drug in his previous episode, the same drug should be used to begin with now. Alternatively, or if information is lacking, haloperidol could be used, beginning with a dose of 5 mg three times daily, with a larger dose, for example 10 mg, at night. The dose would then be adjusted according to his response. As his symptoms come under control, the assessments by the multidisciplinary team that would be appropriate for his diagnosis and background should be arranged. Meanwhile efforts would be continued to establish his family history, and (with his agreement) re-establish contact with his family if his isolation from them is related to his presentation. It might also be necessary to liaise with his employer to ask about recent changes at work, and his level of functioning there, and to do everything possible to keep his job open for him to return to when recovered.

3. His prognosis largely depends on diagnosis but even if paranoid schizophrenia is confirmed, his history of one acute short-lived episode ten years ago, with adequate functioning subsequently, and a second acute episode now, for which he has spontaneously sought help, all point towards a good outcome, particularly if he is compliant with medication. His social isolation, however, is a troubling feature, and unless steps can be taken to reduce it, it may well limit his potential for recovery.

Case 11.1

A 24-year-old man who had previously had one episode of schizophrenia, when he had complained that people were taking note of him in the streets, accusing him of homosexuality, presents at the out-patient clinic. He had an admission lasting six weeks and has been completely symptom free for the last four years. However, over the past year, he has become increasingly anxious and is wary of going out. There is no evidence of psychosis. On further questioning it is discovered that he is shy of going out and mixing, because he thinks that people are looking at him, and he is unable to go into public places. He has no friends and finds it difficult to eat out.

Questions

1. What would you do next?
2. Assuming there is no psychosis and this is social phobia in a shy, introverted individual, how would you outline your management?
3. Behavioural therapy has been of benefit in such cases. How would you plan therapy for such an individual?
4. What drugs would you use?

Answers

1. It would appear from the given information that this patient is suffering from social phobia rather than psychosis. However, the extent of the problem, specific situations and precipitating, perpetuating and ameliorating factors should be assessed. The first time it happened should be explored and he should be taken through a specific occasion when he felt like that. His experience of anxiety (especially the somatic symptoms) and any panic attacks should also be assessed. If it becomes clear that this is social phobia, characterized by blushing, shaking, becoming anxious, unable to talk to strangers or go into situations which may be new,

and unable to eat in public, any ideas of extensive self-consciousness, especially about his appearance, should be looked for. These may be harbingers of a psychotic episode. It is important to assess the extent of any self-medication, especially with alcohol.

2. Having first established the absence of psychotic features or a depressive illness, management would begin by reassuring the patient that he is not suffering a relapse of his schizophrenia and does not require admission. This may in itself be sufficient to relieve some of his anxiety.

Social phobia is best managed using psychological approaches, and in particular behavioural methods, including anxiety management and graded exposure to feared situations. These may be supplemented by cognitive approaches in which automatic negative patterns of thinking are identified and challenged. The initial assessment needs

Case 11.1 decision tree

```
┌─────────────────────┐
│ 24-year-old man.    │
│ Previous schizophrenic │
│ Social phobia       │
└─────────────────────┘
          │
┌─────────────────────┐         ┌──────────────────┐
│ Exclude psychotic relapse │────│ Treat accordingly │
│ or depressive illness │         └──────────────────┘
└─────────────────────┘
          │
┌──────────────────────────────────┐   ┌──────────────┐
│ Differentiate social phobia (newly arising) │──│ Social skills │
│ from avoidant personality (long-standing) │   │ training     │
└──────────────────────────────────┘   └──────────────┘
          │
┌──────────────────────────────────┐   ┌──────────┐
│ Assess self-medication (drugs/alcohol) │──│ Reduce   │
└──────────────────────────────────┘   └──────────┘
          │
    ┌─────┴─────────────────────┐
┌──────────────────────┐  ┌──────────────────────┐
│ Psychological treatment │  │ Drug treatment       │
│  anxiety management   │  │  anxiolytics         │
│  systematic desensitization │  │  antidepressants     │
│  imagery             │  │ may help in short-term │
│  biofeedback         │  │ but high relapse rate │
└──────────────────────┘  └──────────────────────┘
```

to establish whether he is sufficiently motivated to under-take and persist with such treatment, and, if possible, to identify a potential co-therapist among his family or their contacts.

It would also be important to take steps to reduce his social isolation once he becomes capable of interacting with others more freely: to this end, day-centres, social clubs and youth organizations are all potentially useful.

3. The therapy should be planned in collaborative discussion with him. The first step is to set out one or two specific goals of treatment, and a hierarchy of feared situations. The possible psychopathology of anxiety in social phobia should be explained to him. Following this, anxiety management with muscular relaxation and respiratory control can be started, then graded exposure to the dreaded stimulus (also called systematic desensitization).

In addition, positive imagery and bio-feedback methods can be used. Assertiveness training would be developed with modelling, role rehearsal and role reversal. Homework and behavioural tasks can be used to continue the process of learning, positive reinforcement, and change.

4. The drug most often used for social phobias is one of the MAOIs. Phenelzine, 15 mg four times daily, is the recommended dose. Other drugs have been used, especially benzodiazepines and occasionally propranolol, but evidence of benefit is not strong, and relapse rates on discontinuation are high with MAOIs. Since its potential interaction with food is a serious problem, the use of phenelzine should be commenced carefully with regular supervision.

Case 11.2

A 15-year-old boy is referred for psychiatric assessment by a social worker. He has a long history of car thefts and stealing. He had been expelled twice from two schools. He is the oldest of three children—his father, who left home years before, occasionally returns, usually when drunk and hits the patient's mother, who works regularly and does not spend a lot of time at home. The mother describes her son as impulsive, wanting immediate satisfaction, and says that 'He takes after his father.'

Questions

1. What other information would you like?
2. What is your differential diagnosis?
3. Outline your management plan.
4. What do you know of adolescent personality disorder?

Answers

1. More information should be obtained from his previous schools and from the social work department. A detailed history should also be obtained from the mother about the parental marriage as well as the family set-up and the social background. Developmental milestones and academic and social adjustments should be assessed as well as medical history. The patient's attitudes towards his problem, his family and his school as well as his anxieties, can be determined by questioning. His motor development, attention span, level of intelligence and emotional state should be assessed.
2. If this boy's antisocial behaviour is persistent and excessive, as seems to be the case, and is associated with distress on his part or evidence of more generally disturbed personal functioning, then the appropriate diagnosis is conduct disorder. If, however, it is simply a matter of antisocial or criminal behaviour alone, then the relevant label would be juvenile delinquency, though this is a legal category rather than a medical diagnosis and there is much overlap with the socialized sub-type of conduct disorder. Both conditions are much more common in boys than girls, and are associated with low social class, large family size, inconsistent parenting, and a parental history of antisocial personality disorder.
3. A full initial assessment is required, covering the physical and developmental history and mental state examination, and including informant accounts from the mother as well as reports from school on his educational performance, from a

psychologist on his intellectual function, and from the social worker. This would normally be carried out as an out-patient, though occasionally admission to an adolescent unit may be required.

Subsequent management then involves, for conduct disorder, a mixture of family therapy, individual counselling, remedial teaching and provision of alternative outlets for his energy, via youth clubs and outward bound courses. Juvenile delinquency may require management in a forensic setting, such as a Borstal, and may need a firmer and more paternalistic regime. In either case, treatment should be undertaken not in the expectation of a cure, but in an effort to aid maturation and to limit the expression of antisocial behaviour. A high proportion of both groups continue to display personality problems in adulthood.

4. Personality disorders are deeply ingrained and maladaptive patterns of attitudes and behaviour, which are generally recognizable in adolescence and continue through adult life, though often waning in intensity by middle age; and which cause the patient himself, those around him, or society in general to suffer.

By definition, therefore, they may be present in adolescence, though given the adolescent's potential for further maturation and development, it is usually only in retrospect that an adolescent can be given the label of personality disorder. Applying the label at an early age may have iatrogenic consequences, in that an adolescent so labelled may be treated differently, and consequently behave in such a way as to confirm the prediction made of him.

For children, it is better to describe patterns of behaviour in terms of temperament, which, though generally stable throughout childhood, and predictive of some aspects of adulthood, does not carry the implied finality of the term personality.

Case 11.3

A 10-year-old girl who cannot move her right arm is referred. The problem began when, just before her school examination, she heard that her best friend had died in a car accident. She had a similar problem about a year previously when the complaint of numbness in her right arm lasted for three days. She has been examined by the neurologist and the paediatrician who have found no physical explanation of her illness. She is described as a nervous child with very over-involved parents who are very protective of her. She used to bite her fingernails and used to wet herself until three years previously.

Questions

1. What other information would you like?
2. The child tells you that she has headaches and stomachaches and when she is ill her mother looks after her rather than her baby sister. How would you tackle this?
3. What is the prognosis of this child?

Answers

1. The parents and the patient should be interviewed separately to get information on the onset of the present symptoms, as well as the previous episode. The family history and the development of the child as well as the child's current mental state should be assessed. The school should be contacted, with the permission of her parents, to get her school records and find out if she had had any problems there.
2. The phenomenon of somatization (the presentation of psychiatric illness or psychological distress through physical symptoms without organic pathology) may be even more common in children than in adults. Transient abdominal pains and headaches are the commonest symptoms, and are generally dealt with by reassurance from the family practitioners. More worrying is the evidence of conversion disorders producing pseudo-neurological symptoms, as here.

This is much rarer, more persistent and more difficult to treat.

To deal with the recurrent headaches and abdominal pain, in this case, it would be necessary to establish the pattern of relationships between the child, her mother and her sister. If it is true that symptom production is positively reinforced by a diversion of maternal attention from the sister to the patient, this needs to be explained to the mother and tackled along simple behavioural lines.

The symptoms in the right arm, being related to two distressing events (the threat of the impending examination and the loss of the best friend) might best be dealt with by allowing the child to ventilate and discuss her distress, rather than concentrating on the symptoms themselves. This will require the involvement of the parents, who will need guidance and help.

3. Mild, transient physical symptoms of psychological origin are very common in childhood and of little prognostic significance, and as in this case they should resolve. Conversion symptoms have a more variable prognosis, though in general it is worse. It has been reported that, as in adults, a high proportion of those with conversion symptoms go on to develop physical illnesses (Rutter and Hersov, 1985) and some become chronically disabled by their symptoms. The extent of chronic disability is greater if treatment is delayed so that symptoms and patterns of secondary gain become well established.

Reference

Rutter, M.L. and Hersov, L. (1985) *Child Psychiatry: Modern Approachs*. Blackwell, Oxford

Case 11.4

The duty psychiatrist is called to the emergency clinic to assess a distressed 32-year-old man who is asking for help. He says that if he doesn't get help, he is going to kill someone.

Questions

1. How would you deal with the situation?
2. If, after your assessment, you are convinced that he is a psychopath, how would you assess dangerousness?
3. How would you manage him?
4. Give his long-term prognosis.

Answers

1. The most important concern is to assure the safety of other patients, one's colleagues and oneself while conducting the assessment. It should be insisted upon that the patient agrees to be searched for weapons and to be interviewed in a safe room (fitted with an alarm button) in the presence of nursing staff. If he refuses these requests, the police should be called and asked to deal with him initially.

   The next step would be to assess his dangerousness by establishing whether he has threatened or harassed anyone so far, by clarifying the nature of his current distress, and by examination for evidence of psychosis or intoxication with drink or drugs. It would be important to gather as much third party information as possible, to supplement his own account, and the examination findings.

2. It is important, first, to obtain full information about any past history of violence, covering its nature, severity and consequences. Next, the severity of his threat needs to be considered: How determined is he? Does he have a particular victim in mind? Has he made any plans or preparations? Does his current behaviour fit with a previously established pattern? Is there evidence of an escalating series of threats and incidents? Attention should also be directed toward any

recent changes in his circumstances which may make previous equilibrium unstable.

3. It is likely that his threats are related to his inability to tolerate frustration arising out of stressful circumstances: these should therefore be tackled with a crisis management approach, using appropriate members of the multidisciplinary team. He may benefit from a brief crisis admission while the factors causing him distress are tackled; but in general, conventional psychiatric in-patient units have little to offer such patients, and medication is of little or no value.

Over the longer term therapeutic communities (including Grendon Underwood in the prison sector) can lead to changes in behaviour, particularly if the patient is of normal or near-normal intelligence. However, admission to such units is a major step, and for many patients the best long-term management may be through an out-patient service which teaches a problem-solving approach to future frustrations.

4. Antisocial personality disorder, like all personality disorders, tends to improve with increasing age, but good follow-up information is scanty. There is evidence of an increased risk of alcoholism, depression, suicide, and of continuing interpersonal problems even if offending diminishes (Robins, 1966). The best guide to prognosis is the history so far; if this is his first contact with psychiatric services, and he has not yet acquired a forensic history at 32 years of age, his prognosis is probably good.

Reference

Robins, L. (1966) *Deviant Children Grown Up*. Williams and Wilkins, Baltimore

Case 12.1

A 78-year-old man, who lives alone in a flat, is referred by the head of the day-centre that he attends twice a week. For about a month, he has been complaining that another client of the centre has been making homosexual passes at him. On one occasion, this lead to a confrontation between them. He admitted to the centre's occupational therapist (OT) that occasionally he heard the fellow client's voice calling to him: 'Come to me' and that he had been feeling low.

Questions

1. How would you reach a diagnosis?
2. What would your differential diagnosis be?
3. What medication would you use?
4. What is the prognosis of paraphrenias in the elderly?

Answers

1. First, it is necessary to clarify the truth or fantasy of the patient's claims. If, as seems likely, given the source of referral, they are untrue, the mental state of the patient should be assessed, after obtaining a history from him and from the day-centre, his general practitioner and other available sources.

   A likely diagnosis, with these symptoms in this age group, is that of paraphrenia. Initially defined as a well-organized system of paranoid delusions with or without auditory hallucinations existing in the setting of a well-preserved personality and affective response, paraphrenia develops usually in the single person with a premorbid schizoid or paranoid personality. If married, they may have had unsatisfactory relationships and sexual adjustment. They may have sensory deficits of one kind or another, e.g. deafness or cataract. People of lower social class seem to be more vulnerable and sufferers often live in poor inner city housing. Feelings of depressed mood are not uncommon. All these areas need to be assessed to reach a diagnosis.

2. The patient displays paranoid delusions, possible auditory hallucinations, and a lowered mood arising in late life. It would be important to exclude an organically based psychosis by physical examination and appropriate investigation. A psychotic depression is also a possibility, especially if the patient reacts to his psychotic symptoms with guilt and self-blame. Making this diagnosis would require a demonstration of affective changes before the delusions emerged, and would be supported by a family and personal history of previous affective illness, as well as by prominently lowered mood at interview. If in doubt, a trial of antidepressants may be required.

   An acute or sub-acute paranoid reaction to stress is possible but unlikely to arise anew at this age. If the delusional beliefs are circumscribed and accompanied by well-preserved personality and affect, but hallucinations are absent, a diagnosis of paranoia or paranoid state may be made. If hallucinations are confirmed, paraphrenia is the appropriate diagnosis. Paranoid schizophrenia would be a better label if there is evidence of deterioration of personality or affect, or associated first-rank symptoms can be demonstrated (see decision tree).

3. It may be necessary to exclude a primary diagnosis of psychotic depression, or to treat associated depression, with antidepressants. Paraphrenia and related paranoid psychoses require long-term treatment with antipsychotics, probably as a depot preparation. Vulnerability of the elderly to side-effects must always be considered in prescribing these drugs. This particularly applies to anticholinergic effects which can precipitate delirium, postural hypotension, urinary retention and constipation. It is probably better to use thioridazine and trifluoperazine (depending on the degree of agitation) rather than chlorpromazine and haloperidol as more commonly prescribed in younger patients.

4. With or without treatment the condition is chronic, but medication may allow the patient to conduct a reasonably normal life despite continuing delusional beliefs. Abnormal premorbid personality, especially of the paranoid or schizoid

type, poor social support, poor compliance with medication and underlying cerebovascular disease all predict a poor outcome. If there are associated sensory deficits, prognosis can be improved by attending to these (e.g. by arranging the removal of cataracts, or provision of a hearing aid).

Case 12.1 decision tree

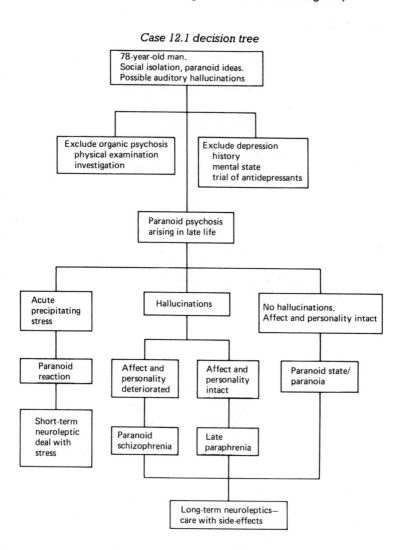

The best prognostic indicator in this patient may be his willingness to continue attending the day-centre, especially if he can be persuaded to accept medication there.

Case 12.2

A young woman brings her 51-year-old mother to the out-patients department because she thinks that her mother has been depressed for six weeks following the sudden death of her salesman husband in a car accident in a different part of the country. Since then, she has become quiet, eats very small amounts and appears to have been crying silently, and on occasions has been irritable. There is no evidence of weight loss. Physical examination shows no abnormality.

Questions

1. How would you proceed?
2. What are the bad prognostic factors in this case?
3. What role do antidepressants have to play in this case?
4. What advice do you need to give to her daughter?

Answers

1. The first question to be established is whether this is a normal grief reaction, or whether there is a superimposed depressive illness. The mother and daughter would have to be seen separately at first to establish the relationship between the husband's death and the development of the symptoms, to enquire about past episodes of depressive illness, and tactfully explore any current suicidal ideation. Morbid preoccupation with worthlessness, marked functional impairment, and psychomotor retardation all suggest an episode of depression complicating the bereavement.

   Next, the amount of support available to the patient and her daughter in dealing with their loss, and its legal and financial consequences would have to be confirmed. Their ability to grieve openly, and to discuss their reaction to their bereavement with each other and with other people, should also be established. If there is no additional depression, but the patient is unable to grieve, she should be offered a fixed number of out-patient sessions to discuss her loss and encouraged in coming to terms with it.

2. Sudden, especially violent, death has been linked to an increased risk of an abnormal grief reaction, because of the lack of opportunity to prepare for the loss, and the consequently greater guilt at things left undone or unsaid. This may be particularly true if the relationship had been an ambivalent one.

Other factors suggesting a poor prognosis, but not applicable in this case, include initial absence of grief, or, conversely, an extreme reaction to the loss (Parkes, 1972).

From the information available, it is difficult to assess this patient's prognosis, but there is little to suggest she is markedly different from most widows, 80% of whom are improved at three months.

3. Antidepressants should be avoided, unless there is clear evidence of a superimposed depressive illness. Their sedative action may delay and inhibit the expression of grief, and they offer a dangerous opportunity if the patient has suicidal impulses. There is no evidence that they accelerate or ameliorate the normal grief reaction. They should be held in reserve until sufficient time has passed to demonstrate the abnormality of this patient's grief, and should only be used in conjunction with psychological approaches, such as guided mourning or supportive psychotherapy.

4. It is important to find out the reasons for the daughter's worry, and why she thinks her mother needs psychiatric help. Once the reasons are available, these should be addressed directly. In addition, comforting the daughter and convincing her that her mother is working through a normal healthy mourning process, which will take time, and will probably resolve without any major consequences, are important factors in the management of this case.

138

Reference

Parkes, C.M. (1972) *Bereavement*. Harmondsworth, Penguin

Case 12.3

A 4½-year-old boy who is not speaking fully is referred for psychiatric assessment. According to the general practitioner, the parents, who are both teachers, noted that their son's motor development was well advanced for his age. When questioned, the parents say that he is the second child in the family, and as an infant he used to express his wants by 'shrieking'. At the age of 2 years he started to speak single words and had no problem in enunciating these words. According to the parents, he is 'really no trouble at all', and is quite happy listening to music and turning the pages in books, of which he has many. He is able to take his models apart and reassemble them without any problem. His physical investigations, including audiometry and neurological examinations have been normal. While the parents are being interviewed, the child is playing with the telephone directory and starts to scream when attempts are made to take it from him.

Questions

1. What questions do you want to ask in order to further your diagnosis?
2. To support your diagnosis are there any physical examinations you would like to carry out?
3. Outline your management plan.
4. Give an outline of long-term outcome of infantile autism.

Answers

1. Questions should be aimed at establishing a clear understanding of the presenting problem and its associated features; and at describing a full developmental history and

account of the family relationships. This should yield sufficient information to distinguish between the various diagnostic possibilities, which include autism (perhaps the most likely), elective mutism, disintegrative psychosis, developmental speech disorder, and childhood schizophrenia.

Elective mutism will be characterized by refusal to speak in some situations (such as school), accompanied by normal speech at home, and is clearly not the case here. Childhood schizophrenia resembles the adult form and is exceedingly rare, though delayed speech may be part of the prodrome. Disintegrative psychosis is also unlikely, in that a period of normal development is followed by loss of (rather than failure to acquire) speech and social interactions, together with disturbances of behaviour and cognitive functions. Developmental speech disorder is typified by a child who appears to understand speech, but whose own speech, though plentiful, is hard to understand because of its abnormal form: again this appears to be unlikely in this case.

Speech disorder is one element of the autistic triad, and as well as sparseness of speech, there may be echolalia, pronoun reversal and a characteristic stereotyped, pedantic use of words and phrases. The parents would be asked about the presence of these features, as well as about the other elements of the autistic triad, autistic coldness (cold relationships with others, including the parents, gaze avoidance, distress at close contact) and obsessive desire for sameness (in clothes, food, toys, etc.). In addition, there may be hyperkinesia, stereotypical motor behaviour and sudden unexplained episodes of anger or fear.

2. There are no physical signs pathognomonic of autism, but observation may reveal the stereotypical motor behaviour sometimes seen. Soft neurological signs are common but non-specific and attempts at physical examination to demonstrate them may provoke the characteristic distress at human contact. Some autistic children appear to enjoy being spun round, and may display whirling movement spontaneously.

3. There is no specific treatment, and medication does not help, except through a non-specific sedating effect for hyperactive children. Management will include work with

the parents and the child. The parents will need support and advice and may benefit from referral to a voluntary agency. Various studies have demonstrated that even with minimal schooling autistic children can make appreciable social and educational gains. Progress is fairly dependent on the child's IQ, which is commonly very low, although this does not appear to be a major problem in this case. A structured educational setting, relevant to the child's cognitive abilities, is important; and the structure can also be used in home-based management. Giving parents direct training at home in the management of behavioural problems has been shown to work. Behavioural treatment involves giving consistent reinforcement for appropriate behaviour and withdrawing attention or positive consequences to help reduce undesirable behaviours. Language skills too can be increased by using consistent reinforcement. Specific behaviour problems such as social withdrawal, self-injury and disruptive behaviour need to be addressed, and may require individually tailored behavioural regimes.

4. The outcome, generally, remains poor, though social intervention has been shown to improve short-term prognosis. In adult life, nearly two thirds of patients may be severely handicapped, thus requiring residential care. Only 15% or so may become independent enough to live in the community and obtain work, though even they continue to show odd behaviour and language problems.

   The prognosis is strongly associated with IQ. A better outcome is also said to be related to acquisition of functional speech before the age of 5 years; mutism indicates a poor prognosis. A small number may regress in adolescence and may need institutional care.

Case 12.4

A 43-year-old woman is referred to the liaison psychiatry clinic by the neurologists. They have investigated her extensively for a number of different neurological symptoms, including aphonia, fainting spells, and blurred vision. All investigations have been normal. She has an extensive past medical history and a very substantial file, having been seen in sucession, over many years, by gastroenterologists, cardiologists, and gynaecologists. She has had an appendicectomy, where a normal appendix was removed, cholecystectomy and a hysterectomy. When you see her she is not very co-operative, and says that she does not understand why she has been asked to see a psychiatrist, since all her problems are physical.

Questions

1. What do you make of this presentation?
2. How would you confirm a diagnosis of somatization disorder?
3. How would you manage her?
4. What role do you think doctors and the structure of the health service play in causing this condition?

Answers

1. The initial suspicion on hearing this history, may be that this woman suffers from Bricquet's syndrome, or somatization disorder. These patients, who are almost always women, are defined in DSM-III-R as presenting with multiple physical symptoms which begin before the age of 30 years and persist for several years. To meet the criteria, patients must show evidence of at least 13 from a list of 35 symptoms, which have not occurred exclusively during panic attacks, and which have caused the patient to alter her behaviour. For each symptom there must either be no organic pathology which might account for it, or, if there is some such pathology, the degree of complaint and functional impairment must be far in excess of that expected from the physical findings. Somatization disorder is the most severe of the somatoform disorders and, through its definition in terms of early onset and chronicity, and its lack of response to treatment, it is more akin to a personality disorder (axis II) than an illness, (axis I). Patients can remain in medical clinics for

years before being identified, if ever, and can undergo numerous costly investigations, surgical procedures, and courses of drugs with little benefit and iatrogenic risks. They are usually very functionally disabled, being unable to work, and in receipt of invalidity benefit. Secondary depression is a common finding.

2. Making the diagnosis is the most important part of management, and requires some care. Patients with somatization disorder rarely give a full past medical history on the first interview, and, where they do give information, they will indicate that investigations had proved abnormal where this is in fact not the case. The best way to document their medical history and therefore confirm the diagnosis is to obtain from the patient a list of hospitals they have attended and then obtain the records from all these hospitals. In this context, the general practitoner's records, as a central repository of hospital out-patient letters and discharge summaries, can be invaluable, and should provide sufficient information to ascertain whether the requisite symptom number has been reached. The fact that *some* investigations may prove abnormal does not discount the diagnosis so long as other criteria are met, for organically based physical symptoms commonly co-exist with symptoms which have no such basis. This effort should not lead to neglect of the psychiatric history and mental state examination, because other conditions, particularly panic disorder, phobias, and depression, commonly co-exist with somatization disorder and are much more amenable than it is to treatment.

3. There is no treatment that is likely to cure her. Management is therefore directed at damage limitation, over a long period, once the diagnosis is made. This will require liaison with her general practitioner and hospital consultants, and an agreed management plan where one doctor accepts responsibly for her overall care. She should be seen regularly, rather than on demand as new symptoms arise. Her complaints should be listened to sympathetically, and she should perhaps be examined regularly, but further investigation should be resisted, and frequent changes of drug treatment avoided. Persistent but not over-bearing attempts

to demonstrate to her the link between psychosocial pressures and her physical symptoms should continue to be made in an effort to change the focus of her attention from her body to other aspects of her life. Any co-existing psychiatric disorders will need treatment in their own right.

4. Somatization disorder appears to be much more common, or at least more commonly diagnosed, in the USA than in the UK. This may be because of lack of interest in the subject in the UK, but it may also be because the structure of the health care system in the USA makes it much easier for patients to gain direct access to hospital specialists, and because there is no comprehensive primary care network in the USA which might identify such patients and prevent them being over-investigated and over-treated. The action of doctors in responding to symptoms by ordering investigations which prove negative are *by definition central* to the diagnosis of somatization disorder—in contrast to any other non-somataform disorder. In that sense the disorder is *per se* iatrogenic: but it is iatrogenic too in the stronger sense that it is *brought about* by several tendencies in doctors' behaviour. These include the tendency to specialize in organ systems, and to react to a symptom with an investigation without considering fully the overall life-long pattern of symptoms, particularly those affecting other organ systems; the tendency to defensive medicine; and the tendency to consider psychiatric diagnosis by exclusion after all physical explanations have been ruled out. It is still considered worse to miss a physical diagnosis by not ordering a test, than to fail to make a psychiatric diagnosis and therefore avoid unnecessary tests.

Reference

Bass, C.M. (1990) Somatisation disorder: Critique of the concept and suggestions for future research. In *Somatisation Physical Symptoms and Psychological Illness*, (ed. Bass, C.M), Blackwell Scientific Publications, Oxford.

Case 13.1

A 28-year-old bank clerk of Trinidadian origin is examined in the casualty department. He was brought in by the police after he smashed the window of a department store in the high street. He had behaved peculiarly and was excited. He shouts at anyone who approaches him to get away from him. He then starts to run around the department and has to be restrained by four nurses. His sister tells you that she had discovered that he had broken off with a girlfriend three months ago, and he started to behave differently soon afterwards.

Questions

1. How would you proceed?
2. What role do life events play in the onset of psychosis?
3. How does the incidence rate of schizophrenia in persons of Afro-Caribbean extraction compare with that of the indigenous population?
4. What is his prognosis?

Answers

1. The immediate priority is to ensure his safety, and that of other patients and staff, as well as of hospital property. It is possible that restraint alone will be sufficient to calm him, so as to allow a preliminary assessment. In order to test this, the nurses could be gradually withdrawn, one at a time (but asked to remain nearby). It is more likely, however, that he will require sedation for continued agitation. There is enough prima facie evidence of mental disturbance to justify this as an emergency under common law, whether he consents or not. There would then be an opportunity to take a history from his sister and, if possible, the arresting police officers. This needs to cover the presenting incident, the recent changes in his behaviour, any past history or family history of psychiatric illness, and any evidence of drug abuse. If he is not sedated, and is able to communicate, it is

important to seek evidence of psychotic phenomena, especially delusions and hallucinations. If simple drunkenness is excluded, various diagnostic possibilities arise, including brief reactive psychosis, schizophrenia, a manic episode, schizoaffective disorder, and a drug-induced psychotic episode. To distinguish between them, to treat him appropriately, and to ensure his continuing safety, he needs to be admitted, probably under Section 2 of the Mental Health Act 1983 (Section 26 in Scotland), and probably to a facility for intensive psychiatric care in the first instance.

2. Brown and Birley (1968), in a controlled study of datable first onset and relapse episodes of schizophrenia, showed that the rate of life events independent of illness events was increased in the three weeks before the onset of acute symptoms in the schizophrenic group. However, these are non-specific events and also occur before episodes of other psychiatric conditions. The association of life events and onset of depression is the most widely researched and shows a clear excess of apparently precipitating life events prior to onset. Brown and Harris' model of chronic difficulties and vulnerability factors is well established and shows that life events may also act as precipitating factors. Vulnerability factors include having young children at home, lacking a confiding relationship, and being unemployed. Loss of mother by death or separation before the age of 11 years was also seen as a vulnerability factor, though not all of these factors have been reported in other studies. Similarly, an increase in life events has been reported prior to the onset of mania, though the evidence is much less clear-cut.

3. Various studies have argued that the rates of schizophrenia are 3–14 times higher in Afro-Caribbean immigrants to the UK compared with the indigenous white population. There are methodological problems with some of these studies (some studies have relied only on admissions, others have not included a control group, and their denominator for calculating the rates has not been very precise), but there has been agreement that Afro-Caribbeans, especially second generation immigrants, are at increased risk. Various explanations, both social and biological, have been suggested for this, including the experience of racial discrimination and

social adversity, increased vulnerability to obstetric complications or viral infections in pregnancy, and differential rates of cannabis abuse. Others have suggested that racial differences do not increase the risk of developing schizophrenia, but do increase the risk of being hospitalized and diagnosed schizophrenic in the event of uncharacteristic behaviour.

4. Commenting on prognosis first requires that a diagnosis be established, and there is insufficient evidence in this case to permit this so far. He and his family will clearly be very concerned about his future, but it is best to avoid discussing prognosis until after a period of assessment. It has been claimed that Afro-Caribbeans are more vulnerable than whites to brief reactive psychosis, with a characteristically sudden onset of florid symptoms and behavioural disturbance, followed by resolution over several weeks, and a

Case 13.1 decision tree

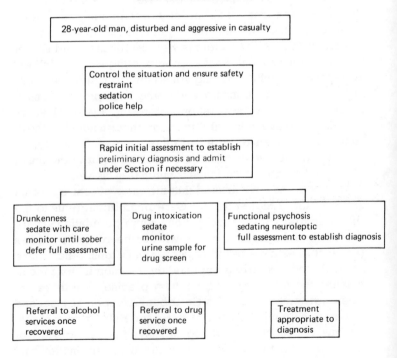

return to full function, but continuing vulnerability to further relapse.

Reference

Brown, G.W. and Birley, J.L.T. (1968) Crisis and life change at the onset of schizophrenia. *Journal of Health and Social Behaviour,* **9,** 203–224.

Case 13.2

A 24-year-old taxi driver appears in the casualty with complaints of 'feeling unreal.' He explains that his body feels as though it does not belong to him, and that he feels unpleasantly detached from himself and his surroundings. He has been working more or less continuously for the last week and on average has managed a couple of hours' sleep every night. He has had periods lasting for several hours when these feelings have gone away but they always come back. He is petrified that he is going mad and says that sometimes he feels like drowning himself.

Questions

1. List your differential diagnosis.
2. What will be your management plans for this patient?
3. What is his prognosis?
4. What medication do you think will help him?

Answers

1. It would appear that he is describing feelings of depersonalization and derealization. These feelings are not uncommon and are quite often related to prolonged tiredness (as may be the cause here), or severe anxiety in normal people. His

reactions suggest that an underlying depressive episode needs to be excluded, and a psychotic state, though unlikely, should be considered, in view of his statement about ownership of his body.

Patients often find it very difficult to describe their experiences of depersonalization and derealization, and may revert to metaphor, as this man has. Care needs to be taken to differentiate these metaphorical descriptions (such as: 'It feels *as if* my body is not my own') from descriptions of somatic hallucinations or delusional beliefs (such as: 'My body *is* not my own').

Depersonalization and derealization phenomena also occur in anxiety neuroses (especially with phobic or obsessional features) and drug intoxication states, as well as dissociative disorders and, occasionally, organic conditions like temporal lobe epilepsy. Rarely, they may occur in isolation from other primary diagnoses.

2. The initial assessment should involve a sufficiently thorough history, mental state examination and physical examination to exclude or confirm the primary diagnoses listed. If, as seems likely, the symptoms are merely the result of tiredness and sleep deprivation, then he should be reassured that, distressing though they are, they are not in themselves serious and will resolve with sufficient rest. His reference to drowning himself indicates that assessment of his suicidal intent is mandatory, and arrangement or provision of appropriate levels of observation and support, if he feels suicidal, is a priority in management. Otherwise, the management of depersonalization is management of the underlying primary diagnosis.

3. If there are no underlying physical or psychological causes, his prognosis is good if he is able to rest and rearrange his work so that he can sleep sufficiently. If depersonalization is the result of some other condition, then its prognosis is that of the underlying disorder. In rare cases of depersonalization syndrome, the symptoms may become chronic and cause long-term distress.

4. No drugs are specifically indicated for depersonalization and derealization, and where the symptoms are isolated, as in the result of sleep deprivation or the rare depersonaliza-

tion syndrome, they are ineffective and best avoided. Where the symptoms arise as part of a primary diagnosis, they should respond to treatment appropriate for that diagnosis.

Case 13.3

A 13-year-old boy who lives in a group home for the mentally handicapped has recently had an increased frequency of epileptic fits, which had been under control for several years. He had been in the group home for five years and attends activities regularly. His family come to visit him and he is generally no problem for his carers.

Questions

1. Outline your assessment.
2. What would you do?
3. What do you understand by the term 'normalization'?
4. What are the long-term sequelae of anti-epileptic drugs?

Answers

1. Epilepsy is particularly common in mentally handicapped patients and the prevalence rate increases with severity of brain damage and intellectual retardation. The increase in the number of fits could be due to a number of reasons. Full background information would need to be obtained on the extent of mental retardation and epilepsy, his functioning and any recent changes in the environment. Previous investigations, the current dosage of medication and the serum levels of drugs should be reviewed.

   Serum levels which are now low but previously therapeutic could explain his increased fit frequency, and could be due to changes in compliance, physical illness affecting the gut and decreasing absorption, a failure to increase the dose in line with his continuing growth (especially now he is in the pubertal age), or induction of liver enzymes by other drugs. All these possibilities should be enquired into. If the serum levels are still therapeutic, then his increased fits could be simply due to physiological changes arising at puberty, or to interaction with other drugs or alcohol, or to underlying nutritional deficiencies. In addition, social pressures and psychological problems, particularly anxiety, might be implicated and should be enquired after, as should any changes in pattern of sleep, diet or exercise. Occasionally, fits may have a very specific environmental stimulus, as in reflex epilepsy. It would therefore be important to obtain from his carers and family a full description of the pattern of his seizures, in an attempt to identify any specific triggers.

2. If the initial assessment identifies possible causes for the increased fits, then these can be attended to directly, by stopping any interacting drugs or by advising his carers appropriately. If, as may well happen, no specific cause can be found, it might first be worth increasing the dose of anticonvulsant, if there is room to do so. If this fails, then changing to or adding another drug is the next step. This needs to be done carefully: there should be a period of overlap during changeover, followed by careful withdrawal of the first drug; and, if the two drugs are to continue, a combination should be chosen where drug interaction and enhanced toxicity are not major risks. It is best to limit treatment to one drug if possible, and certainly no more than two. Throughout this period attention should still be directed at identifying any underlying psychological and social problems which might explain the change, and his carers should be asked to monitor the frequency and circumstances of his fits to try to clarify any pattern.

3. Normalization, a concept pioneered in Sweden, basically means creating an existence for the mentally handicapped as close to normal living conditions as possible. The mentally handicapped carry three burdens—insufficient skills, rejection by society, and awareness of their limitations and differences. Thus, normalization basically requires efforts to ease these three burdens. The aim is to make the lives of the handicapped as normal as possible by appropriate training

to improve their skills, mobilization of social resources, and reducing their self-awareness of difference by offering housing, training and work within the community rather than in a separate institution.

4. The anti-epileptic drugs have varied pharmacology and no generalization will cover them all. The older drugs, phenobarbitone, phenytoin and primidone, as well as causing drowsiness and ataxia in the short-term, tend to produce deficits in concentration, memory, psychomotor skills and other cognitive functions in the long-term. These are less of a problem with the newer drugs, such as carbamazepine and sodium valproate. In addition, phenytoin in particular has undesirable effects on the appearance, causing acne, hirsutism and gum hyperplasia. Like all drugs, anti-epileptics carry the risk of rashes and, more rarely, blood dyscrasia and hepatotoxicity, but there is little evidence of increasing risk with long-term treatment.

Case 13.4

A general practitioner requests the assessment of a 3-year-old girl who is diagnosed as having Down's syndrome. She is an only child of professional parents in their mid-40s, and her mother has been feeling depressed lately.

Questions

1. How would you approach them?
2. Outline the kind of support you would wish to offer and how long for?
3. What is the prognosis for the child?
4. Would you advise admission to a mental handicap hospital?

152

Answers

1. It should be assumed that the general practitioner has already informed the family about the impending referral. The parents should be sent a letter offering an appointment—either as a home visit or in hospital.

   There appear to be two issues here: the child's future management and the mother's depression. It would be best to direct the assessment towards the former first. Since the child has previously been diagnosed, there should already have been a full multidisciplinary assessment, including a developmental history, tests of functional capacity, and an overview of how the family have been coping. It is unlikely, but not impossible, that the child has slipped through the net and never came into contact with available services, in which case the initial assessment needs to be set up now. It is more likely that aspects of the child's assessment now need to be repeated, to address any new problems that have emerged in the child's behaviour.

   The mother's depression is best assessed by an indirect approach initially. She should be asked: 'Has all this been getting you down? How badly?' This would then lead into a fuller assessment of her current mood and how it affects her ability to care for her child. It may well be that her depression is the major element in the current presentation, and so the focus of therapeutic attention needs to be moved away from the child and towards the mother.

2. The prognosis depends very much on the nature of any previous contact the family may have had with support services, and the extent of the child's handicap.

   If the parents had not been prepared for the arrival of a child with Down's syndrome, they may still be in the process of grieving. It would be worth checking if the mother had received any antenatal counselling or amniocentesis. Often counsellors, independent of obstetricians and paediatricians, offer the service. The parents usually go through phases of shock, reaction, adaptation and orientation. It is in the latter phase that they begin to organize, seek help and information and plan for the future of the child. Hence, it is possible that that is why they are here now. Their needs are best met by provision of regular help and guidance. It would be advisable to see them regularly, initially for 4–6 sessions, along with a colleague—a social worker would be ideal—to assess and improve their knowledge of Down's syndrome. The aim is to support and educate them, and set up whatever long-term support may be necessary for their child's special needs. Following the initial sessions and assessment of their needs and their responses, it may be decided to offer a similar number of sessions again. Sometimes an open-ended contract is useful, whereas at other times fixed number sessions may be indicated. Home care may be available through the social worker. Teachers and psychologists may need to be involved. Some authors have recommended parent workshops. Home teaching may be necessary.

3. Like all children, those with mental handicap continue to develop, and are likely to have a range of different needs and capacities relative to their peers at different stages in their growth and development. Nonetheless, the overall level of current handicap is the best guide to the level of future handicap, and the parents need to be advised accordingly. The majority of children with Down's syndrome are moderately or severely handicapped, but a few can eventually function at a level sufficient to permit independent adult living. In general, children with Down's syndrome display fewer problems with temperament and behaviour than those with comparable levels of handicap from other causes.

Associated physical illness is common, including congenital heart disease, intestinal abnormalities, chest infections, leukaemia and thyroiditis. The more severe forms of these illnesses usually present in infancy, but milder forms may emerge later in development. An early onset dementing illness of Alzheimer's type is very common, occurring in over 90% of those over 40 years of age, and leading to death in the fifth decade.

4. Admission to a mental handicap hospital would not be advised. All aspects of assessment are best conducted in a community setting, and in-patient care is likely to be needed only if there are severe behavioural problems not responsive to other management, or major psychiatric

illness is superimposed. Occasionally admission may be requested to establish control of associated epilepsy, or on an intermittent respite basis, to relieve the parents of the burden of care, especially if the mother has a depressive illness. Nearly all mentally handicapped children under 16 years old live at home, including 70% of those with severe handicap.

Case 14.1

A 29-year-old man is admitted to the ward for assessment. His IQ is said to be around 60, and he has been living in a group home for the mentally handicapped. For the previous two weeks, he has been rather aggressive and has hit out twice at the staff. He explains this by saying that the voice of his late grandfather told him to do so. His behaviour prior to this episode had been completely normal. He has been on no medication at all during his stay. There is no family history of psychiatric illness.

Question

1. How would you assess him?
2. What would be your management of this case?
3. Is there a relationship between mental handicap and psychiatric disorder?
4. What is his prognosis?

Answers

1. As much information should be gained as possible about the onset of his illness and his premorbid functioning, from the staff at the group home, the family, the general practitioner and any other available source. It would appear that the patient is borderline handicapped, so it should be possible to assess his mood, abnormal experiences, and aggressive impulses via a thorough mental state examination as for a patient of normal IQ. However, observation of his behaviour on the ward may well be of greater relative importance than for other patients: this may take the form of a chart measuring the antecedents, circumstances and consequences of the particular aspects in behaviour of concern—in this case the aggression.

   Mental handicap and organically based psychiatric illness commonly occur together; he therefore needs a full physical examination in which any neurological signs are compared with those demonstrated at earlier developmental assessments. Investigations should include the usual blood count and biochemical screen, together with a urine drug screen, it may well be that he is manifesting an idiosyncratic reaction to his first use of cannabis or other drugs.

2. It is first of all essential to establish a diagnosis. In this case there is evidence of an acute change in behaviour, with auditory hallucination giving instructions. This constitutes prima facie evidence of a newly presenting psychotic illness which might be affective, schizophrenic, organic (especially related to epilepsy), or drug-induced.

   A period of drug-free assessment (as outlined above) is advisable to establish the diagnosis, providing his behaviour is not too disturbed.

   Once diagnosis is established, the basic principles of management are the same for the mentally handicapped as for other patients. Antipsychotic drugs should be used in much the same way, with more attention to their epileptogenic potential and extra-pyramidal side effects. The staff at the group home may need to be educated about the patient's illness and the importance of medication, allowing him to be gradually re-introduced there as soon as his condition allows.

   Once the acute phase of his illness is past, he will require long-term supervision, on a day-patient or out-patient basis, or, preferably, by a community psychiatric nurse in liaison with the doctor prescribing his continuing medication. If his illness leaves him with deficits in addition to his mental handicap, he may well require an individually tailored rehabilitation programme, making use of occupational therapy and sheltered workshops.

3. There is a complicated interaction between mental handicap and psychiatric disorder. Mental handicap is stigmatizing, isolates the patient (often physically) from society and limits the scope of social interactions with others: all these factors may precipitate psychiatric illness. Alternatively, psychiatric illness and mental handicap may have a common cause, which might be genetic or some underlying organic brain disease. In addition, mental handicap has a powerful pathoplastic effect, modifying the cause and mani-

festations of psychiatric illness. Together, these and other factors lead to psychiatric disorder of all kinds being commoner in the mentally handicapped. Rates for schizophrenia and manic depressive illness both reach 5—6%, and neurotic conditions are correspondingly more common too. Behavioural disturbances, such as head-banging and other forms of self-injury, may not have the status of psychiatric disorder but are common, occurring in up to 40% of severely retarded children, and can pose serious management problems.

4. Mental handicap often modifies the course and presentation of psychiatric illness, leading to difficulties and delay in diagnosis. Furthermore, the deficit of the illness and the handicap may have a mutually magnifying effect. For these reasons the prognosis may be worse than for an otherwise comparable patient of normal intelligence. However, good prognostic factors here include his relatively high IQ and premorbid level of functioning, the lack of a family history, and the acute presentation.

Case 14.2

A 60-year-old grandmother is referred to the out-patient clinic by the general practitioner. Since the birth of her first grandchild, five years previously, she had become a 'frequent attender' at the surgery, presenting at least once a week. Her first symptom was pain in her joints which responded initially to anti-arthritic agents. She then developed headaches and pains all around her body, which have not improved with any medication for any more than a few weeks at a time. She has been concerned about her heart and her health generally after her brother was admitted with a stroke and diagnosed as having diabetes.

Question

1. What would you advise the general practitioner?
2. What do you understand by the term 'hypochondriasis'?
3. How would you deal with the family who do not feel that their mother needs to see a psychiatrist?

Answers

1. Any advice to the general practitioner would depend upon the general practitioner's purpose and expectations in making the referral, and upon the confidence with which underlying physical causes have been ruled out by examination and investigation. This might need to be established by discussion with the general practitioner in advance of seeing the patient, if it is not clear from the referral letter.

It may be that the general practitioner wants nothing more than the exclusion of a formal psychiatric illness, particularly depression, underlying the patient's somatic presentation, followed by treatment if any is required. This would require a full history and mental state examination, and if depression is confirmed, a combination of pharmacological treatment (antidepressants) and psychosocial measures. Throughout, it would be important not to neglect adequate physical assessment and investigation; a substantial proportion of patients with physical symptoms referred to psychiatrists later develop evidence of underlying physical illness (Slater, 1965).

Many patients who present with physical symptoms without organic pathology have no formal psychiatric illness, although there may be clear evidence of a relationship between the symptoms and social stresses, life events or mood states. If the general practitioner is requesting help with management, it is not sufficient simply to refer the patient back having excluded psychiatric illness: instead attention should be directed at the postulated causal role of psychosocial factors, via simple social measures or formal psychological treatment. Cognitive behaviour therapy has shown itself to be of value in these patients.

2. Hypochondriasis refers to a transient or permanent pattern of preoccupation with health and bodily symptoms, a tendency to misattribute bodily sensations to the effects of illness, and a habit of repeated medical consultation and reassurance-seeking. It may arise in primary psychiatric disorders, such as depression, or, transiently, following adverse life events. Alternatively, it may be an enduring aspect of a patient's character, more akin to a personality trait (or even disorder) than an illness or response to stress.

3. If the views of the patient's children have little effect upon her willingness to accept the referral and treatment, it may be unnecessary to do anything more than note them and respond only if she fails to make progress. If, as is more likely, their views are strongly expressed so that she is influenced by them and therefore less likely to engage fully in treatment, they need to be tackled directly. This might best

Case 14.2 decision tree

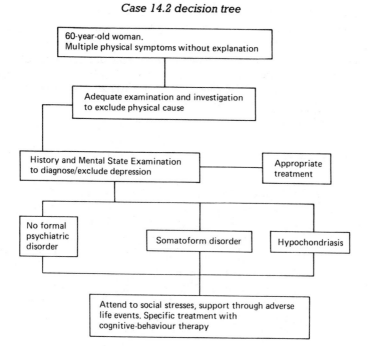

60-year-old woman.
Multiple physical symptoms without explanation

Adequate examination and investigation
to exclude physical cause

History and Mental State Examination
to diagnose/exclude depression

Appropriate
treatment

No formal
psychiatric
disorder

Somatoform disorder

Hypochondriasis

Attend to social stresses, support through adverse
life events. Specific treatment with
cognitive-behaviour therapy

be done in a family meeting, where they have an opportunity to air their concerns, and there is an opportunity to explain that referral to a psychiatrist does not imply 'madness' or 'weakness in the head' on the part of the patient. The best approach might be to point out that the frequent visits to her general practitioner have not ceased, despite many different physical treatments over the last five years: now might be the time for a trial period of psychiatric treatment, over, say, three months. If she is no better after that, then she could be referred back to her general practitioner. In any case, close liaison will be maintained with her general practitioner. An important part in management, if the family are closely involved with the patient on a day-to-day basis, would be to educate them about how to respond when she refers to physical symptoms in their company. Attempts at psychological treatment may well fail if the patient receives a lot of reassurance from her family between sessions.

References

Slater, E.(1965) Diagnosis of Hysteria. *British Medical Journal*, **i**, 1395–1399

Warwick, H.W. and Salkovskis, P.M. (1990) Hypochondriasis. *Behavioural Research and Therapy*, **28**, 105–117.

Case 14.3

A general practitioner has asked for an assessment of a 55-year-old man who gets very irritable. On detailed questioning it is discovered that his irritability is to do with his inability to remember things; especially at work, he forgets where he had kept his files and papers and then starts to shout at his secretary. The company doctor thought that he was depressed due to increased pressure at work following a takeover of his company. About 25 years ago he had been treated with ECT for what his family describes as 'depression'. On examination, he begins by shouting: 'I am not mad', then calms down and agrees to be interviewed.

Questions

1. What questions do you need to ask to reach a diagnosis?
2. What investigations would you order?
3. What is the distinction between dementia and pseudo-dementia?
4. What advice would you give the family?

Answers

1. A full history of present complaints will be the starting point, and a complete and well-documented past history is essential. This would include asking about the mode of onset and form of presenting symptoms in the previous admission, along with previous medical history, previous and current medication, premorbid personality and functioning and relevant family history. Past and present levels of alcohol consumption need to be documented.

   The patient's mental state must be assessed with particular emphasis on cognitive performance and mood. A detailed cognitive assessment is mandatory, and should cover orientation, memory (registration, immediate recall, and remote memory), concentration, as well as tests of verbal memory, naming ability, mathematical skills, and so on. Any new physical symptoms suggestive of underlying organic illness should be enquired into in detail.

2. In addition to obtaining third party information from the family and other sources about his premorbid functioning and onset of present symptoms, and a full physical examination, physical investigations such as a full blood count with erythrocyte sedimentation rate, a biochemical screen, serum B_{12} and folate, and syphilis serology should be carried out. Hypothyroidism may be diagnosed by low levels of serum thyroxine and raised TSH levels. A chest X-ray is needed to exclude underlying bronchial carcinoma. Alcohol abuse

may be suggested by a macrocytosis with folate deficiency and raised liver function tests.

3. The distinction can be difficult to make, yet it is important that every effort is expended in the attempt. Compared with an organic dementing illness, depressive pseudomentia is commonly of more abrupt onset, with a higher frequency of past history or family history of depressive illness. Patients are usually more distressed by their cognitive deficits, and complain of them more. They more often make 'don't know' responses than errors, and there may be much variability in their cognitive performance on testing. Specific defects, such as dysphasia or dyspraxia, strongly suggest an organic illness. Where these features do not help in differentiating between the two, a therapeutic trial of antidepressants may be of benefit.

4. Initially, the family should be told that the patient needs a period of investigation and assessment in order to establish a diagnosis. They should be allowed to ask questions regarding particular diagnoses they might be concerned

Case 14.3 decision tree

about. At the assessment stage diagnosis and prognosis should not be discussed in detail.

If depression is confirmed on the diagnosis, the family should be reassured that a full recovery can be expected, though it may take some time, and is dependent upon adequate medication, which they can help oversee. It may be that one or more family sessions may be necessary to address any stresses within the family which precipitated or maintain the depression.

If, on the other hand, the diagnosis is dementia, then a full discussion of the prognosis is required, at an appropriate time. This should cover the expected decline in the patient's capacities, the need to make legal and financial provisions, and the likely need for home support. The family should be told about services, such as home helps, meals-on-wheels, district nursing, day-centres, and voluntary agencies, and should be reassured that they will be helped in their efforts to care for the patient.

Reference

Lishman, W.A. (1987) *Organic Psychiatry*, 2nd edn, Blackwell Scientific Publications, Oxford, p. 410

Case 14.4

A 42-year-old woman telephones to ask for an assessment of her 6-year-old daughter as an emergency. On questioning, she reveals that the main problem is bed-wetting. Her daughter has been dry for six months and has started bed-wetting again, and the mother says she cannot cope with 'all this nonsense'. You initially try to resist the 'emergency' but then arrange to see her the following morning in the out-patients clinic. The mother and daughter are 20 minutes late because they couldn't find a parking space.

Questions

1. What kind of questions do you want to ask?
2. What do you make of the mother?
3. Outline your management plans.
4. What role will medication play in managing this child?

Answers

1. The pattern of bed-wetting first needs to be established. Is the daughter wetting the bed every night, or only occasionally? Is she incontinent during the day? Has she regressed to her previous pattern of bed-wetting, or is the current pattern new? Any recent changes in home circumstances need to be considered: there may be recent conflict between the parents, or the child may be attending school for the first time.

    The background needs to be explored by way of a full developmental history, a description of the family history and family relationships, an account of previous medical problems and physical systems review, which may reveal evidence of urinary tract infection.

2. The mother appears to be demanding in approaching the psychiatrist directly rather than via her general practitioner, in insisting on an emergency appointment and then arriving late, and in seeking help for what she describes as 'nonsense'. This suggests that what motivates her approach are her own anxieties and needs, rather than concern for her child's welfare. If the girl is her only child, born when the mother was 36 years old, she may well be a career woman who is now finding intolerable the additional pressures of motherhood. This would need to be explored, albeit tactfully, through questions about the mother's job, her relationship with her husband, and her general satisfaction with life.

3. If initial assessment confirms, as appears to be the case, that this is an instance of primary enuresis (there not having been one year of continence before enuresis re-emerged) complicated by the mother's anxiety, then investigation to exclude organic causes, particularly urinary tract infection, diabetes, and epilepsy is required.

A behavioural approach is then the best initial management, in which the child is rewarded (using a star chart) for dry nights, rather than punished with scolding for episodes of incontinence. It will be important therefore to try to modify the mother's attitude, and, through explanation that this is a common problem with no blame attached, to reduce the child's guilt.

If these measures are insufficient, an enuresis alarm (the bell and pad method) may help, via conditioning and other learning mechanisms.

With these simple approaches, about 75% of children will be dry within three months.

4. Drugs, especially tricyclic antidepressants, have been used, but the side-effects can be troublesome and relapse rates are high, and there is a risk of accidental poisoning. However, due to their simple quick action they may be indicated for immediate short-term effect, through their anticholinergic action.

Case 15.1

A 52-year-old chronic schizophrenic man, who has been in a maximum security hospital for 18 years following an index offence of grievous bodily harm, has been referred by the regional forensic consultant to the catchment area psychiatrist for general psychiatric opinion. It would appear that the man is 'ready for rehabilitation into the community'.

Questions

1. How would you proceed with assessing him and what particular areas would you wish to clarify?
2. Outline your rehabilitation plans.
3. What are the chances of him re-offending?
4. What would be your main worries about having him on your unit?

Answers

1. It should be arranged to assess the patient without undue delay. Appropriate multidisciplinary team members should be assembled to review his case notes and discuss him with members of his current clinical team, particularly the nursing staff. His progress in recent years, his current mental state, and especially his views and wishes for the future, should be discussed. The likely problems that may have arisen as a result of institutionalization should be assessed, including any limits in his ability to care for himself, and his interactions with female staff or other females, especially if he has been on a male ward. More information is required about any family support that may be available and how the family might become involved in the management plan. After assessing his needs, it has to be made absolutely certain whether the facilities for meeting those needs are available.
2. Since he has been in hospital for 18 years and is described as chronic schizophrenic, it would appear that some degree

of rehabilitation should have started long ago. His progress thus far needs to be ascertained, and, in order to build on that progress, relevant team members (for example the occupational therapist) should be encouraged to contact their counterparts. Systematic rehabilitation would include assessing and improving his activities of daily living and then moving on gradually to more independent living. His medication would need to be monitored as well as his social and interpersonal skills. Initially, the patient may be encouraged to be transferred on a trial leave rather than full transfer.

3. If there had been only one crime 18 years ago and there haven't been any further aggressive outbursts, it would appear that he is unlikely to re-offend. However, the nature and circumstances of the index crime need to be borne in mind, especially such factors as his mental state at the time and the precipitants of his offence. If his offence was psychotically driven and there has been no recent evidence of positive psychotic symptoms, then he is unlikely to re-offend, provided compliance with medication can be assured.

   His behaviour since admission to hospital may help to clarify the continuing risk: any evidence of violent outbursts or threats towards other patients or staff will be a cause for concern, as will the fact that his admission was so long. Also relevant will be his willingness to accept some degree of responsibility for his offence and good evidence of willingness to comply with treatment in order to prevent any future relapse.

4. Possible problems will include matching local facilities to his needs, especially accommodation, occupation, medical and social supervision; and concerns about his recent behaviour. Any attached publicity may be another source of worry.

Case 15.2

A 48-year-old male architect is referred for psychiatric assessment because he feels frightened and has started to see the ghost of his wife every night. His wife died suddenly three months ago at the age of 42 years of a heart attack. He has a 15-year-old son, who is away at a boarding school. When you see him, he appears dishevelled, unkempt and sad. He bursts into tears when you ask about the circumstances of his wife's death.

Questions

1. What do you think is happening here?
2. How would you manage him?
3. When does mourning become abnormal?
4. How would you manage someone with abnormal or pathological mourning?

Answers

1. It appears most likely that the patient is going through a process of mourning following his bereavement. It would be essential to rule out any underlying depressive episode, which would be clarified by taking a detailed history of his symptoms and their duration. The way people manage the process of mourning depends not only on their own personality but also on their previous experiences of loss, their relationship with the deceased, their social support network, and general cultural attitudes. Differentiating normal and abnormal mourning may be difficult, and even normal mourning may require a period of support and psychological help from medical services. In this case it appears that visual hallucinations have caused the current presentation. These are relatively common in the bereaved, and are usually hypnogogic in nature.
2. He needs to be reassured that hallucinations of the type he describes are not evidence of mental illness, that they occur

frequently in the aftermath of bereavement, and they subside with the passage of time.

If an associated depressive illness is excluded by history and mental state examination, then he should be managed as a case of normal mourning. It is best to avoid medication if possible, as it may interfere with the psychological adjustment required, though a short course of benzodiazepines may be required for severe sleep disturbance. He needs sympathetic supportive listening which will allow him to ventilate his feelings regarding his wife's death. This will be particularly important if his relationship with her had been ambivalent. Any tendency to resort to excessive alcohol use should be monitored and discouraged as counter-productive. If he is socially isolated, as it appears, then attempts to increase his social support during this difficult period will be needed. He should be encouraged to return to work. It is

Case 15.2 decision tree

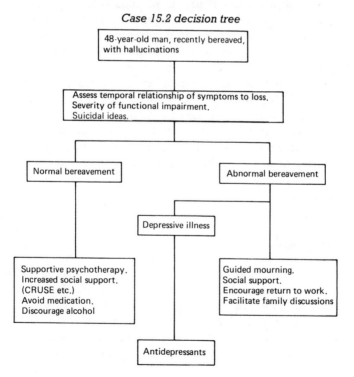

worrying that his son, who is presumably also distressed, is away from home: it may be wise to liaise with the school doctor or housemaster about his son's adjustment to his loss.

3. Abnormal grief may be distinguished from normal mourning by its prolonged duration relative to the norms for that culture, especially where it is associated with marked functional impairment, a morbid preoccupation with worthlessness, or psychomotor retardation. Feelings of loss and sadness persisting for many years, but not associated with these other features, are not in themselves abnormal.

4. Where bereavement is abnormal it is most often complicated by an episode of major depression, which will require appropriate antidepressant treatment. This will be of limited benefit unless psychological and social aspects of management are pursued in addition. If bereavement results in social isolation, as is often the case, putting the patient in contact with a support group, such as CRUSE, may be the most important aspect of management. Guided mourning is a psychological treatment conducted along behavioural lines, in which the patient is gradually encouraged to expose themselves to evidence of their loss. The underlying model is that the patients avoid such exposure (e.g. by not attending the funeral, or not visiting the grave) and that the avoidance perpetuates the continuing distress.

Patients are therefore encouraged to sort through and discard the deceased's belongings, and to visit the grave, in an attempt to break the cycle of avoidance and continued distress.

Case 15.3

A 58-year-old Indian man presents in the out-patients clinic with six month's history of erectile dysfunction. He had been married for 35 years and his wife died three years ago. They did not have any children because his wife had had tubercular salpingitis. Sexual life, according to him, was satisfactory. He arrived in the UK in 1959, and has been running a corner shop for the last 15 years or so. It transpires that he has been out twice with his white neighbour, who is 62 years old and widowed. On the second occasion, when they attempted sexual intercourse, he failed to have an erection. He maintains that he has 'no sexual hang-ups' and believes that there is something physically wrong with him.

Questions

1. How would you assess him?
2. What physical investigations are necessary?
3. What psychological methods of treatment would you use?
4. What do you know about intrapenile injections of vasoactive drugs?

Answers

1. Erectile dysfunction may be due to physical or psychological factors or a combination of the two. In a middle-aged male, presenting for the first time with erectile dysfunction, since he is presenting alone, his history has to be relied on. He should be asked about the onset of the problem, whether he is able to obtain erections at all, specifically morning erections, his ability to maintain an erection, his anxieties, his fantasies and possible precipitating and perpetuating factors. He should be asked to describe his last successful sexual encounter and his last attempt. His orgasmic and ejaculatory difficulties should be assessed. In addition, more should be found out about his sexual drive, masturbatory patterns, especially after his wife's death, and any other worries that he may have. He will need a thorough medical history and examination, as well as appropriate investigations to exclude physical causes; and a psychiatric history to rule out psychological illnesses, particularly depression.
2. It is important to take his perception of physical problems seriously. Basic haematological investigations including full blood count, packed cell volume (PCV), serum folate and vitamin B_{12} should be carried out. Particularly important, given his age and ethnicity, is a fasting blood sugar level to

exclude diabetes. A thyroid profile, liver function tests, urea and electrolytes, serum testosterone, gonadotrophins and prolactin may be indicated. In some centres, penile plethyomographs are used as a routine.

3. The treatment strategy would depend on the possible aetiological factors. Any psychological treatment must be accompanied by full treatment of physical abnormalities.

The first step is education. It is possible that this patient is suffering from guilt about starting another sexual relationship, especially with a white woman. Since this patient is single and the dysfunction may have happened on only one occasion, he may need no more than simple reassurance and education. However, if the problem has been present frequently with different partners, a variety of behavioural techniques developed by Masters and Johnson are the treatment of choice.

Treatment is short-term and focused on symptoms, with the couple being given a series of exercises, hierarchically arranged, to work through between sessions. The emphasis is on mutual pleasure rather than performance, and on reducing anxiety by improving communication and by gradual desensitization.

Case 15.3 decision tree

Psychodynamic psychotherapy is occasionally used, but there is little evidence of its effectiveness for these problems. If sexual dysfunction is aggravated by more extensive marital disharmony, then couple therapy may need to accompany the more specific sex therapy if it is to be successful. Cognitive therapy has also been used for managing such cases.

4. Intracavernosal injections of vasoactive drugs, such as papaverine, have been used for about 10 years to treat impotence. The treatment is clearly effective, but local side-effects of bruising, fibrosis and priapism are troublesome. The latter needs treatment in a casualty unit, and patients need to be informed about the risk and given information sheets to show to treating doctors. Priapism is treated by withdrawing blood from either corpus cavernosum and then injecting phenylephrine (while monitoring blood pressure).

There have been several potentially fatal cases where papaveretum was dispensed instead of papaverine, so care needs to be taken in writing the prescription and warning the patient to check the drugs.

Reference

Gregoire, A. (1992) New treatment for erectile impotence. *British Journal of Psychiatry,* **160**, 315–326

Case 15.4

A 14-year-old girl, the youngest of four sisters from a high achieving family, is referred for psychiatric assessment. Her parents say that she has lost 9 kg in the last three months. She eats only small amounts because she says eating causes abdominal pain. She weighs 32 kg and her height is 1.58 m. She started her periods a year ago and after the first three periods she has not had any. The other sisters are 16, 18 and 22 years old— all outgoing, gregarious types. Both parents are professionals and are very busy with their lives.

174

Questions

1. Outline your assessment.
2. What would you look for in physical examination?
3. What physical investigations do you need done?
5. What is the prognosis?

Answers

1. Because of the age, sex and mode of presentation, the most likely diagnosis is anorexia nervosa. The immediate focus in this patient is to assess her impaired nutritional state and associated physical complaints and complications. A thorough history of presenting symptoms is essential. Specifically, any refusal to maintain normal body weight, loss of weight through various means, fear of becoming fat and a body image distortion should be elucidated. She may be quite secretive about her eating and, in view of her abdominal pain, her physical state should be assessed. The history should be elicited from her parents too. It is vital to establish trust and rapport with them—they may be feeling guilty about having failed as parents or not recognizing her symptoms earlier. Symptoms of depression, anxiety or an obsessive compulsive disorder must be ruled out, and in this context, family history of affective disorder may give a clue to the problem. A developmental history from the patient's family will enable an assessment of the patient's autonomous functioning to be made.

2. A thorough physical examination is essential to rule out any physical disease, especially since the patient is complaining of abdominal pain. This may be due to chronic grumbling appendicitis, giardiasis, regional enteritis, Crohn's disease or a number of other causes. On physical examination, the physical stigmata of eating disorders should also be ruled out, e.g. muscle wasting, lanugo, brittle hair, bradycardia, hypothermia and parotid enlargement, and tooth damage from self-induced vomiting— though the latter two are associated with bulimia nervosa.

Primary panhypopituitarism may need to be considered, though it is unlikely in this case because the patient has already had periods. Occult malignancy, Addison's disease, diabetes mellitus and other endocrine disorders may all need to be excluded.

3. A full blood count, biochemical screen, liver function tests, thyroid function tests and cortisol and gonadotrophin levels should be conducted. A skull X-ray and brain scan may be essential if there are endocrine abnormalities and a pituitary lesion is suspected.

4. If a diagnosis of anorexia nervosa is confirmed, and she is left untreated, her prognosis is poor, with a mortality rate of 10% or so. With treatment, approximately one third of patients recover completely, one third improve but continue to display some abnormal eating, and one third are unchanged or worse. Factors indicative of a poor outcome include a long history, considerable weight loss, poor relationships with family and peers, as well as older age at onset and male sex. Bulimic features at presentation also suggest a poor outcome.

Sample cases for MRCPsych I examination

Case I

A 35-year-old Muslim woman with four children was admitted to the ward three weeks ago. Her problems arose six weeks previously when she refused to go to India with her husband. She was noted to be behaving bizarrely, giggling and laughing to herself while reading the Koran. She says that she did not need any sleep and that she had been given a healing gift by the gods to cure the world. She felt that she did not need any clothes and had been running out of the house with the youngest child to 'wash him in the rain'. Episodically she was seen talking to herself and a week before admission she switched on all the lights and electrical appliances in the house simultaneously. She could not explain why. She started smoking the day before admission and had not washed for days. She had a similar episode lasting two days five years ago which resolved without treatment.

Both her parents have had psychiatric admissions in India and both had ECT, although the exact diagnosis is not known. One of her sisters is said to have been treated with antidepressants. Four other siblings are alive and well without any problems.

She was born in India and came to the UK aged 6 years. At school she was an average student who got along well with peers and teachers. She did not gain any qualifications, and left school to start work as a packer, a job she had held since then. At 19 years of age she entered an arranged marriage to a man who came from India to join her. He is a mini-cab driver now aged 36 years, and they have four children aged 14, 13, 11 and 9 years. Initially he used to be verbally aggressive towards her because she held a job and went out of the house. This settled down when the first child was born. They live in a four-bedroomed council house with her parents and the children.

On mental state examination she is a slim, small Indian woman in Western clothes who speaks softly in excellent English. Her hair is dishevelled and her appearance unkempt, but there are no abnormal movements. She shows adequate eye contact though poor rapport. She is distractible but not overactive. Subjectively she says she feels 'very happy', but objectively looks very preoccupied, distracted and suspicious. She shows flight of ideas and is complaining that people are plotting against her family because she has a four-bedroomed council house. She can clearly hear the voices of these people talking about her. Occasionally a voice talks to her and says: 'Don't sleep'. No formal thought disorder is apparent and her orientation is intact.

Questions

1. What is your differential diagnosis?
2. How would you elicit auditory hallucinations?
3. What is the difference between pseudohallucinations and real hallucinations?
4. What is flight of ideas?
5. What other symptoms would you look for to make a diagnosis of a manic episode?

Answers

1. The most likely diagnosis is a hypomanic episode in view of the history of bizarre behaviour and delusions of grandiosity of acute onset, the examination findings of distractibility, flight of ideas and possible elation, the probable family history of affective illness and the past history of a similar but self-limiting previous episode. However, because of the paranoid features and second person auditory hallucinations a diagnosis of paranoid schizophrenia needs to be considered. First rank symptoms may occur in up to a fifth of manic patients, but they tend, along with delusions, to be less persistent than in schizophrenia.

2. In clinical situations care must be taken in framing the questions to elicit them. The phrase used in the Present State Examination (PSE) (Wing, Cooper and Sartorius, 1974) is: 'I should like to ask you a routine question which we ask of everybody. Do you ever seem to hear noises or voices when there is no one about, and nothing else to explain it'? Also: 'Do you ever seem to hear your name being called?' This

needs to be clarified further by using subsidiary questions like: 'Do you hear noises like tapping or music? Does it sound like muttering or whispering? Can you make out the words? What does the voice say? Do you hear several voices talking about you? Do they refer to you as he/she? What do they say? Do they speak directly to you? Do they give you orders? Do you obey? Do they call you names? Can you carry out a two-way conversation with them? Do you see or smell anything at the same time as you hear the voice? What is the explanation? Are these voices in your head or do you hear them through your ears'?

3. A hallucination is a sensory misperception occurring in the absence of an external stimulus. Hallucinations have a quality similar to ordinary sense perception, and are located in the external world rather than the mind or the 'mind's eye'. They are not subject to conscious control. Pseudohallucinations are perceived as arising in the mind as a particularly vivid form of mental imagery beyond conscious control, or in an alternative definition, as hallucinations where the subject recognizes the absence of an external stimulus.

4. A patient displaying flight of ideas will experience and verbally express a sequence of thoughts in which there is rapid progression from one subject to another, via connections which are understandable but inappropriate in the context, such as rhymes, punning and abrupt references to environmental cues. Communication is impaired because such patients can rarely complete one train of thought before moving to another, and then another, in rapid succession.

5. As well as the symptoms this patient displays (grandiosity, with related persecutory ideas, distractibility, flight of ideas and possibly elation) manic patients may show irritability and transient depressive features. They are often overactive and can appear to have a lot of energy, though this is usually not well-directed. There is usually a decreased need for sleep and increased desires for sex and food. Flight of ideas is often associated with pressure of speech. Caution and restraint may be swept away and insight lost, so that those afflicted indulge in reckless driving, extensive gambling, spending sprees and sexual indiscretions whose consequences return to haunt them when they recover.

182

Reference

Wing, J.K., Cooper, J.E. and Sartorius, N. (1974) *Measurement and Classification of Psychiatric Symptoms*. Cambridge University Press, Cambridge

Case II

A 64-year-old man was referred to the hospital by his general practitioner and is currently an informal patient. Six weeks before admission, he went to the general practitioner with a persistent dry cough and a chest X-ray revealed a lesion in his left lung. He coped well with investigation at the local general hospital, but two weeks before the admission he was told that the lesion was a slow-growing bronchogenic carcinoma, and he then became very anxious. He also felt depressed, with loss of appetite, anorexia, anergia, initial insomnia and early morning awakening, feelings of hopelessness and worthlessness, and a fear of death. He admits to having had serious suicidal thoughts, and he says that he has decided that he would collect his tablets and take them as soon as he is left alone.

In 1987, following the death of his wife and 29-year-old son in a car crash, he had become very anxious and depressed and was admitted to a psychiatric hospital for six-months when he was treated for depression with ECT and psychotherapy. He later had a brief admission lasting three weeks when his mother died three years ago. One of his aunts who had a drink problem and attended Alcoholics Anonymous, had killed herself following a diagnosis of breast cancer.

His father died when he was 10 years old and his mother brought him up. He was born and raised in Galway as the youngest of eight siblings. He did his schooling in Ireland before coming to the UK aged 18 years. He started work as a labourer and has worked with the same construction company ever since. He is currently working as a foreman. His employers have been very supportive and helpful. He describes himself as a worrier, with fishing as as his hobby. He goes to the local pubs occasionally and drinks no more than two pints a day.

On examination, he appears gaunt, wasted, unshaven and slow in his responses, though his talk is coherent. He appears depressed and at one point bursts into tears saying that he didn't want to die even though death didn't mean anything to him. He admitted to a fear of the future and felt that he had let his dead wife down. He showed poor concentration and poor memory but was orientated to time, place and person.

Questions

1. How would you differentiate between endogenous and reactive depressions?
2. How would you assess suicidal risk?
3. How will you differentiate between anxiety and depression?
4. How do you assess psychomotor retardation?

Answers

1. Various classifications have been proposed for depressive disorders, of which the distinction between endogenous and reactive depression is one of the most enduring. The terms suggest that the distinction is based purely on the presence or absence of an obviously precipitating stress or life event, but they have also been used to denote symptom patterns, so that endogenous depression is characterized by prominent biological symptoms and reactive depression by prominent anxiety features. The two types have also been claimed to differ in prognosis and treatment response, so that endogenous depression responds well to physical treatment with drugs and ECT and resolves fully but tends to relapse, while reactive depression responds poorly to physical treatments and tends to run a chronic course with variations in severity. The validity of the distinction has been challenged, and other classifications proposed, such as: psychotic versus neurotic, primary versus secondary; uni-

polar versus bipolar, and pure depression versus depressive spectrum disorder.

2. The risk of attempting or committing suicide is correlated with many factors relating to the individual's social and demographic groups, medical and psychiatric history, and the degree of suicidal intent exhibited. The patient's age, sex and social class, and employment and marital status are all connected with suicidal risk, but not specifically enough to give more than general guidance in a particular case. More closely connected with risk are: a history of current serious physical illness; a current or previous psychiatric illness, particularly depression, schizophrenia and alcoholism; previous attempts at suicide; and degree of social support. The most specific guidance on the short-term risk of suicide in someone who has attempted or is contemplating it, comes from an assessment of suicidal intent. This requires detailed but tactful enquiry into the extent of any preoccupation with self-harm, the degree of planning undertaken, the method chosen, the adoption of precautions against rescue or discovery, the leaving of notes or other warnings and the reaction to the failure of the attempt.

3. Distinguishing anxiety and depression can be difficult. In addition the agitation of depressed elderly people may often resemble an anxiety state. These often occur together, and each may give rise to the other. In very general terms anxiety is a response to perceived threat, and depression a response to perceived loss, but threat and loss are often intermingled. A man who is made redundant after 15 years not only loses companionship, and self-esteem, but faces threats to his security; he may well present with an equal mixture of anxiety and depression. Anxiety symptoms often arise in a primary depressive illness, and resolve with it, and conversely depression may be a response to the limitation imposed by an anxiety neurosis, such as agoraphobia. In attempting to distinguish the two, the main aim should be to decide whether they are co-occurring, in a mixed neurosis, or whether one is primary to the other, since this will determine the best treatment approach.

4. Psychomotor retardation is a psychomotor disturbance often seen in severe depression. An affected individual will

talk, think and move much more slowly than normal. There may be long pauses before the subject answers questions and each word follows very slowly after the one before. Occasionally, the patient may stop answering altogether and may need to be reminded before starting again. Patients may sit abnormally still, and when required to move often pause for a long time before starting. When severe, psychomotor retardation is better described as depressive stupor. Assessment therefore needs to cover the speed of the patient's movement, speech and thought processes.

Case III

A 34-year-old Irish man has been brought to the hospital on Section 136 by the police. He had been so agitated, confused and disorientated in a taxi he ordered, that the driver had been obliged to stop and radio the police for help. He had told the driver that the taxi was crawling with ants, and asked the police to take him to the nearest pub because he needed a drink. Subsequently, it becomes apparent that he was sacked from his job as a pub manager two weeks previously and had to leave the flat which came with the job. He had disappeared for a time, apparently sleeping rough, but a week previously he had been taken to the police station where he was seen by a police surgeon who did not think that he was ill in any way.

Three years previously he had a motorcycle accident when he had been unconscious for three days and also had a fractured mandible. The patient denies any drink problem, but does say that he is often accused of it.

The youngest of four siblings, he was born and brought up in Ireland. He did two 'A' levels and decided to pursue business studies. He did the first term of a three year course and gave it up because he was working in a pub. Subsequently, he has been sacked from four pubs—all on the account of being drunk on duty. He had been involved in three driving offences and lost his licence a year ago. He describes himself as 'sensitive', but denies any close heterosexual or homosexual relationships.

There is no past or family psychiatric history. His father is said to 'like his pint'. Both parents are retired and live some distance away. The patient has no contact with them.

On examination, he is dishevelled and unkempt, fidgety and restless. He appears to be visually hallucinating and occasionally scratches various parts of his body because 'the insects are biting me'. He says he feels fine in himself, but objectively he appears somewhat perplexed. His attention, concentration, registration and short-term recall are poor. He appears disorientated to time, place and person. He does not appear to be thought disordered.

Questions

1. What questions do you need to ask him to get a drinking history?
2. How would you test his short-term memory?
3. What are the psychological disabilities associated with alcohol abuse?
4. What are the physical sequelae of alcohol abuse?
5. How would you define alcohol units?
6. What do you make of his references to ants and biting insects?

Answers

1. Taking an alcohol history is a necessary part of any psychiatric assessment, but if heavy drinking is suspected, the questioning must be more extensive and more detailed. Alcoholics and heavy drinkers can be very evasive and inaccurate when asked to quantify their consumption, so their answers should not necessarily be taken at face value. The best way to approach the subject is to go through a typical drinking day, working backwards from the evening. The points to establish include the time of the first drink, whether this is taken in response to withdrawal symptoms, the total number of units of alcohol consumed on an average day, and the preferred types of drink and settings for drinking.

The patient should be asked how he feels on waking, and what happens if he goes without alcohol for a day or two, to confirm the presence of withdrawal symptoms. Once an accurate picture of the current level of drinking is established, attention can move to the history and consequences of this drinking pattern, via such questions as: How long have you been drinking at this level? Has it affected your health? Has anyone advised you to cut down for health reasons? Were you able to? Has your drinking affected your work, or your family life? Has it brought you into contact with the law?

It may be necessary to get third party information from the patient's family, friends, or employers (if the patient agrees) to confirm these details of the history.

2. Short-term memory, which lasts up to about five minutes, is to be distinguished from immediate recall (seconds) and long-term memory (minutes to decades). Deficits in each are identified by appropriate bedside tests and have different clinical implications. Short-term memory is commonly tested by asking the patient to commit to memory a name and address, and then recording the accuracy of recall when asked again after five minutes, during which they are given different tasks. Alternatively, a standard sentence such as one of those introduced by Babcock (e.g. 'One thing a nation must have to be rich and great is a large secure supply of wood') can be used. A normal person should require no more than three repetitions to retain the sentence and recall it accurately. Visual memory can be assessed in similar ways by showing the patient a diagram and asking them to copy it from memory both immediately and after a five-minute delay.

3. The common psychological disabilities associated with alcohol abuse include acute intoxication, dysphoria, blackouts, personality deterioration, sexual problems, irritability and aggression; and more psychotic phenomena such as delirium tremens, alcoholic hallucinosis and morbid jealousy, as well as cognitive deficits which may amount to dementia. Heavy drinking itself can produce a very depressing effect on mood and the drinker may become a prey to all sorts of doubts, miseries and suspicions.

Rates of both non-fatal deliberate self-harm and completed suicide are raised in alcoholics, 15% of whom kill themselves eventually. Acute intoxication with alcohol in patients who are not alcoholic is a common accompaniment of drug overdoses, and can complicate their management.

4. Alcohol exerts damaging effects on many body systems, either by direct toxicity, or its association with nutritional deficiency and heavy smoking. The gastrointestinal tract is commonly affected. Fatty infiltration, hepatitis and cirrhosis of the liver, oesophageal varices, gastritis, peptic ulceration, and pancreatitis are all relatively common. The nervous system can be damaged both centrally (in the Wernicke-Korsakoff syndrome, cerebellar degeneration and alcoholic dementia) and peripherally, with peripheral neuropathy occurring in up to 10% of cases. Anaemia, cardiomyopathy, and neoplasms of the oesophagus and the lung and upper airways are all associated with alcoholism, as are tuberculosis and pneumonia. In addition, alcohol is a prominent risk factor, through ataxia or drunken brawling, for trauma and accidents, particularly head injury.

5. A unit of alcohol is a standard measure, equivalent to about 8 g of pure alcohol, allowing comparisons between different drinks. For example, a can of ordinary beer contains 1.5–2 units, a can of strong lager up to 4 units, a pint of draught beer 2 units, a glass of wine 1 unit and a bottle 6 units, and a bottle of spirits about 30 units.

6. It seems that he may be experiencing visual or somatic hallucination, or even both. To clarify this it is necessary to ask him whether he can see the ants and insects, or whether he feels sensation on his skin which he attributes to them. The former is the more likely possibility if, as seems to be the case, he is developing delirium tremens, which commonly involves frightening visual illusions and hallucinations, often of small animals which may be brightly coloured. If he is instead reporting a bodily sensation 'as if' ants were crawling on his skin, then this may be an example of *formication*, which is occasionally found in schizophrenia, but has a particular association with abuse of cocaine.

Case IV

A 42-year-old Afro-Caribbean man was first admitted 15 years ago with what he describes as hearing 'tormenting voices'. He was put on medication which he took for six months and then stopped because he went back to his parents' country of birth. He was apparently well until his return to the UK six months ago, when he became suspicious and again started to hear voices which were tormenting him. These voices could be heard through his ears and were talking about his actions and behaviours. He heard them all the time and was feeling frightened because for the previous week they had been saying that he had to be killed. He had not been able to sleep and had taken to smoking cannabis in order to relax. He believed that the MI5 were after him because he had seen a message to that effect on the television screen. He also knew that people from the secret service had been following him around and that his telephone was bugged.

Apart from the one previous admission, he denied any other psychiatric contact. There is no positive psychiatric history in the family. Both his parents are dead. He has no contact with his ex-common-law wife, who had three children by him, having lost touch with them when he left the country, and he is now socially isolated, living in a bed-sit.

He describes himself as a shy, quiet individual who likes to spend time by himself. He avoids the company of white people because he expects them to make racist remarks. He has a few black friends. He was born and brought up in the UK and went to school here. He did poorly at his studies and had no close friends, but he got on well with the teachers. There is no relevant medical history. He has two younger brothers—one of whom is in prison following an attempted robbery. The other brother works as a car mechanic and the patient has no contact with him.

At interview, the patient is dressed neatly, appears shy and has little eye contact. He smiles inappropriately, has a blunted affect, and appears slowed down. He acknowledges hearing 2–3 voices outside his head, which talk about him and occasionally threaten him, but which do not appear to be related to his mood. He says that he would feel fine if the voices went away.

He keeps looking over his shoulder and is somewhat edgy and defensive on initial questioning, but more forthcoming later. He is convinced that the radio and television are talking about him and that the whole world knows his secrets. He admits to feeling unwell and agrees that he is better off in hospital.

Questions

1. What is your differential diagnosis?
2. How would you assess him for thought insertion, thought withdrawal, thought broadcast and thought echo?
3. What is a delusion?
4. How might you classify delusions?
5. What is the difference between an idea of reference and a delusion of reference?
6. How would you assess insight?

Answers

1. This man is displaying third person auditory hallucinations (a first rank symptom), paranoid delusions and blunted affect, with evidence suggesting a schizoid premorbid personality. The most likely diagnosis is schizophrenia. However, his current use of cannabis makes a drug-induced psychosis another possibility, if it can be established that he was using cannabis before his symptoms began. The use of other drugs should also be excluded. We lack information about his level of functioning for the fifteen years between admissions, but if he functioned well and was symptom-free, schizophrenia would be somewhat less likely, and other possibilities, such as psychogenic psychosis or atypical psychosis should be considered. Finally, an organically-based psychotic illness should be excluded by a full history, physical examination, and appropriate investigations.
2. Thought insertion, thought broadcasting and thought withdrawal are all examples of thought interference, in which the individual has abnormal experiences of thought ownership. The experiences can be difficult to describe and are

often surrounded by delusional elaboration, so assessment is not easy. Patients should first be asked whether they experience any interference in their thought processes. If they do, they should then be asked further whether they experience thoughts, which are not their own, being put into their head by some external agency (thought insertion); whether they are aware that thoughts are broadcast via radio or television, or can be heard directly by others (thought broadcasting); or whether they experience the abrupt removal of their thoughts by some outside force (thought withdrawal). When severe, thought withdrawal is like a sudden emptying of the mind, and brings to a halt any train of thought or conversation the patient is engaged in. This is known as thought blocking.

Thought echo is somewhat different, in that, although the patient's thoughts are not subject to interference, an hallucinated voice repeats them aloud in the manner of an echo. All these symptoms are suggestive of schizophrenia, but none are pathognomonic.

If the patient reports any of these experiences, it would be important then to clarify any delusional beliefs he holds in relation to them, by asking him to whom the thoughts belong if they are not his own, and who does he believe is responsible for the interference in his thinking? Why are they doing it? How does he know? How has he responded?

3. A delusion is a false belief, held firmly despite contrary evidence, and out of keeping with the patient's cultural background. It is held with unshakeable conviction which is entirely disproportionate to the evidence on which it is based, and it cannot be modified by reasoned argument or disconfirmation through experience. Delusions are often imbued with great personal significance, and can lead to dramatic changes in behaviour. Very occasionally a delusion may be true in the sense that the content fits the facts but the logic behind it is flawed: for example, a man who believes that his neighbours and the police are in league against him may respond by playing music very loudly, to drown out the voices he hears, so that his neighbours eventually do complain to the police, who then pay him a visit.

4. Delusions can be classified in various ways, and the most common distinctions are those made on the basis of content or theme. Thus, delusions refer mainly to persecution, hypochondria, jealousy, grandiosity, religion, nihilism, worthlessness, or other themes. Delusions may be primary (or autochthonous), arriving fully-formed *de novo*; or secondary, being elaborated around some other experience such as a hallucination; a normal perception which seems to have great significance (delusional perception); an abnormal mood of foreboding (delusional mood), or a normal memory which has subsequently acquired significance (delusional memory). Occasionally delusions may be shared by more than one individual, as in induced psychosis or *folie à deux*.

5. A patient with ideas of reference may complain that he feels that people in public places take too much notice of him. If they look in his direction, it feels as if they are staring at him, and if they talk to each other, it feels as if they are talking about him.

Although preoccupied and distressed by these ideas, the patient can recognize that they are not based in fact, and that the feeling of being watched or spoken about arises within him. In this sense, ideas of reference are a type of overvalued idea, and are to be contrasted with delusions of reference, in which the patient believes with certainty that he is being stared at or spoken about, or, more dramatically, mentioned in newspapers, on television and on the radio. The references are usually persecutory in nature, and may be linked to an elaborate delusional system.

6. Although assessment of insight is part of every mental state examination, there is little agreement on what is meant by the term. When used in its crudest sense, it can simply denote whether the patient agrees with his doctor that he is ill and in need of treatment: but it is better to think of it as the degree to which a patient is aware of his own mental condition. It is not, as the distinction between psychosis and neurosis suggests, an all-or-none phenomenon, and it cannot be established by asking just one question. It encompasses several elements, including the degree to which a patient sees his experience or behaviour as abnormal; the degree to which the patient sees that abnormality as evidence of

illness, and the degree to which the patient is seeking or will accept treatment for that illness. Each of these elements needs to be enquired into with specific questions, if insight appears impaired.

Case V

A 23-year-old barmaid presents with a two-month history of worry and tension. She had been working until two months previously when she saw a murder in her pub, in which two men got into an argument and one stabbed the other. One of the men had subsequently threatened to harm her if she reported the matter to the police. However, somebody else rang the police who managed to arrest the culprit. Following this, she started to have nightmares, was unable to concentrate, and lost her sex drive. This led her boyfriend to leave her because she was refusing sex. In addition, she discovered that her cat had been run over in a freak accident, though she believed that it was done on purpose, 'to teach her a lesson'. She was unable to pay her rent because she was not working and her landlord was threatening to evict her. She felt overwhelmed and she wanted to die 'to escape all this'. She had felt shaky, with palpitations, sweaty palms and a dry mouth and was unable to mix with people. She was now frightened of leaving the house. She felt low in mood but her sleep was not disturbed. She was eating more than usual and had gained 6 kg in weight in two months.

She is the youngest of three children, her parents are in their mid-fifties and she has very little contact with them. There is no family history of psychiatric illness. She described her childhood as deprived, because her father was often unemployed and her mother had to do cleaning jobs. She is not close to her siblings. She was an average scholar and worked as a shop assistant for three years after leaving school. She was made redundant and since then has been working as a barmaid off and on for three years. She denies any alcohol or drug abuse. She describes herself as nervy and a worrier. She can't stand loud noises and gets very anxious when under pressure. She has never sought help before, always managing to cope.

On examination, she is a small, neatly dressed woman with appropriate responses to questions. She appears anxious and tremulous and becomes tearful when talking of her cat and the murder. She acknowledges that she is avoiding going out because she is frightened that she would faint in public. She denies any suicidal ideation and shows no evidence of abnormal experiences or abnormal behaviour.

Questions

1. Summarize this presentation and suggest your differential diagnosis.
2. Define phobia. What do you understand by the term 'phobic avoidance'?
3. What is a life event?
4. What role do life events play in the genesis of depression?
5. What do you understand by the term 'free-floating anxiety'?
6. How would you differentiate between 'trait anxiety' and 'state anxiety'.

Answers

1. A 23-year-old woman with anxiety traits in her personality presents for the first time with a two month history of physical and psychological correlates of anxiety, lowered mood, and agoraphobic features following two traumatic events. There are no psychotic phenomena and few biological features of depression. The diagnostic possibilities include, in the ICD-9 classification, an anxiety state, a phobic state, a neurotic depression, or an adjustment reaction with predominant features of anxiety. In the DSM-III-R classification the possibilities include agoraphobia without a history of panic disorder, adjustment disorder with anxious mood, or perhaps post-traumatic stress disorder. There is insufficient information to distinguish definitely between them, but the most appropriate diagnosis may well be an adjustment

disorder or reaction. She does not appear to meet the criteria for generalized anxiety disorder or major depression.

2. A phobia is a fear of a particular object, activity or situation, which persists despite being recognized by the patient to be irrational, in that it is out of all proportion to that which is feared. It is beyond voluntary control, cannot be reasoned away, and leads to avoidance of the feared situation.

   Phobic avoidance is the behavioural limitation imposed by a phobia. Its nature depends on the phobia concerned: in agoraphobia, patients stay at home because they fear having a panic attack or fainting in a public place; in animal phobias, they may avoid public parks in case they come across the feared animal, and in social phobia they avoid social gatherings of all kinds. The avoidance, at its extreme, can be very incapacitating, because patients avoid anything where they perceive even a small risk of encountering the object of their fear. Avoidance is a potent factor in maintaining phobias, and the essence of behavioural treatment of phobia is to gradually expose patients to the object they fear while preventing avoidance, until they habituate and the avoidance response is extinguished.

3. Life events are transitions in an individual's life which either constitute major losses (divorce, bereavement); pose major threats (serious illness); impose additional responsibilities (marriage, childbirth); or are a cause of uncertainty and anxiety (moving house). There has been much research to suggest that events of this type occur more commonly in the period preceding the development of many kinds of illnesses, both physical and psychiatric, than would be expected by chance. This is particularly true of depression. However, there are many methodological problems inherent in this research, and it is clear that the majority of people who experience such events do not develop depressive disorders or other illnesses, so, important though they may be, life events do not by themselves explain the aetiology of these conditions and other factors must operate too.

4. Life events and the genesis of depression are said to be correlated, but the relationship is not a simple one. The two could simply co-exist by chance or through some non-specific association; or the direction of causality may be

reversed, so that depression causes poor performance at work and home, leading to the sack, rather than vice versa. Research has tackled these problems by defining the events carefully, using a 'contextual approach' and considering only events clearly independent of any mood change. By these methods, an excess of life events has been shown in the months before the onset of depressive disorder. Paykel (1978) demonstrated that the relative risk of developing depression increased sixfold in the six months after experiencing markedly threatening life events. For attempted suicide, the risk was sevenfold and for schizophrenia twofold. Loss or exit events are said to be more related to depression than neutral or positive events.

An alternative model suggests that rather than simply increasing the risk of depressive illness, life events only bring forward in time the onset of an illness: this can be estimated as the 'brought-forward-time' which generates an estimate of the severity of the event in the question.

5. 'Free-floating anxiety' refers to the experience of the physical and psychological symptoms of anxiety when they occur without being triggered by or directed towards a particular stimulus. Patients with free-floating anxiety are likely to be anxious at all times, to varying degrees, and to express a wide range of fears and apprehensions, in contrast to phobic patients, who are anxious only when exposed to (or anticipating exposure to) a feared stimulus.

6. State anxiety is anxiety experienced at a moment in time, as assessed from a cross-sectional viewpoint, whereas trait anxiety is a tendency to anxiety in a wide variety of different circumstances, and is assessed from a longitudinal viewpoint. A patient who says 'I feel anxious now, in this situation' is displaying state anxiety: while one who says 'I often feel anxious in those circumstances and others like them' is displaying trait anxiety. The two are not mutually exclusive.

Reference

Paykel, E.S. (1978) Combination of life events in causation of psychiatric illness. *Psychological Medicine*, **8**, 245–53

Sample cases for MRCPsych II examination

Case 1

An 82-year-old man who is currently attending a day-hospital for the elderly is seen for psychiatric assessment. His wife was present with him, and from the two of them it is established that he had undergone a brief psychiatric admission five months previously and had attended as a day-patient subsequently. The admission had been prompted by his experience of visual hallucinations, seeing threatening figures in and around his house. Shortly before admission he became very agitated, claiming that the figures were carrying guns and threatening his life. His wife had struggled to cope, with the help of her general practitioner, but admission was required when his agitation became extreme. There had been no previous similar episodes, and this was his first psychiatric contact. Both his parents had died in middle age without any evidence of psychiatric history, but one younger brother had spent many years in a long-stay psychiatric institution, although the nature of his illness was not clear. In addition, one cousin had had repeated psychiatric admissions, during which he was said to 'hear voices'.

The patient had generally been fit and well throughout most of his adult life, although he suffered a serious leg fracture when serving in World War II, and now needed two walking sticks because of secondary arthritis. His vision had deteriorated in the last three years, because of bilateral cataracts. One of these had been removed with some improvement in visual acuity on that side, and he was awaiting surgery to the other eye. In addition, he had bilateral conductive deafness, but could communicate clearly by using a hearing aid.

He had lived all his life in South London, apart from his war service in the Far East. Neither he nor his wife were aware of any particular problems during his childhood and adolescence, and he reported that, although he enjoyed the companionship of his school friends, he was not at all academic. He had left school at the age of 14 years to take up work in the local bakery, where he remained until conscripted. On his return from the army, he found work as a delivery driver in a variety of companies until his retirement at the age of 65 years. He had married at the age of 23 years and his wife was clearly close to and supportive of him. They have three children who live nearby, and who visit regularly.

He described his personality as a quiet home-loving man who enjoyed family life, and his wife concurred with this description.

He says that since his admission he had been taking 'little white tablets' and was convinced that these had helped him sleep, but were not responsible for the departure of the threatening figures. His wife took a different view, clearly attributing the resolution of his presenting symptoms to his admission and continued treatment with medication.

On mental state examination, the patient is found to be a carefully dressed, elderly man who is co-operative throughout, who carries a white stick and wears a hearing aid, and who displays no abnormal movements. His speech is slow and rambling, but not abnormal. He does not appear depressed, and reports no sleep disturbance or changes in appetite. Although he does not now display any delusions, hallucinations or agitation, he can clearly recall the experience of seeing a gang of men carrying shotguns in his front parlour, threatening him and his wife. He remains uncertain whether they were really there, or whether they were somehow products of his imagination. No deficits are demonstrable on cognitive testing of his attention, concentration, memory, and orientation.

Questions

1. Summarize this presentation and give a differential diagnosis.
2. What factors are associated with paraphrenia?
3. If you had been asked to see this man on a domiciliary visit when he first presented, how would you have managed him?
4. How would you use anti-psychotic medication in elderly patients?
5. What prognosis does paraphrenia carry?

Answers

1. An 82-year-old man with no past psychiatric history, but an apparently positive family history of psychotic illness, presents with five-month history of visual hallucinations, and secondary agitation and delusionary elaboration. He has sensory impairment with poor vision and hearing, but is cognitively intact. His presenting symptoms resolved soon after admission and treatment, and he shows no current mental state abnormalities.

   The most likely diagnosis for a psychotic illness arising anew in late life on a background of sensory deficits, is paraphrenia. This is a relatively rare condition which may represent the mode of presentation of schizophrenia in late life, or it may be a separate condition. It shares many features with schizophrenia, but is differentiated by the relatively good preservation of intellect and personality. An important diagnostic possibility to be excluded is an organically based psychotic illness, and this patient requires a thorough physical and neurological examination, as well as investigation with baseline haematology and biochemistry, chest X-ray, and probably a CT scan, to exclude an underlying organic curable condition. Occasionally, depressive psychosis in late life may present with atypical features such as those, demonstrated here, but the lack of prominent mood symptoms would go against this suggestion.

2. Paraphrenia is associated with female sex, a family history of schizophrenia and a variety of factors which all act to increase social isolation. Affected patients are commonly unmarried, or if married commonly childless. Their underlying personality is often of the suspicious, paranoid or schizoid type and they frequently live in almost reclusive conditions. In addition, they are commonly further isolated by sensory defects, most notably impaired hearing in up to a third of patients. Visual impairments also occur, but less frequently. In addition, cerebrovascular disease is found more commonly in these patients than control groups.

3. At his presentation, this man and his family were in crisis, and his diagnosis was unclear. It would therefore be best to arrange a period of admission to allow full assessment and a

diagnosis to be reached, and to give his wife some respite from looking after him. It may well be necessary to use a Section of the Mental Health Act in order to do this. The admission period should be used to exclude organic causes of his condition, to institute pharmacological treatment, and to set up an appropriate network of continuing support to be available on discharge. Paraphrenia is a chronic condition requiring more or less indefinite treatment and supervision. It is therefore important to try to establish a maximally effective drug regime early on, and to keep side-effects to a minimum so as to reduce non-compliance. It would be expected that such treatment might reduce his agitation, but may not completely abolish his symptoms. Once his agitation has settled sufficiently, trial periods of leave overnight and weekends at home should be arranged, and then he should be transferred to day-patient status, once it is clear that he and his wife are able to cope again. An occupational therapy assessment should be undertaken while he is an in-patient, so that a personally tailored programme of occupational therapy could be instituted, and continued as a day-patient. It would be necessary to liaise with his general practitioner regarding his continued drug treatment, and with his ophthalmologist regarding his anticipated eye surgery. Finally, if he and his wife were having continuing problems managing at home, he may well need a home assessment and liaison with home-help and meals-on-wheels services

4. In general, elderly patients are more sensitive than younger adults to most side-effects of anti-psychotic medication, and some of these can be particularly serious. Hypotension leading to dangerous falls, and hypothermia are both dose-related effects likely to arise with short-term treatment, extra-pyramidal symptoms are more common in medium-term treatment than in younger patients, and in the long-term tardive dyskinesia (also see p.81) is a particular problem in the elderly. For these reasons, careful consideration should be given to the prescription of anti-psychotics to elderly patients, but some, like this man, clearly need them, and they should not be needlessly withheld. It is best to prescribe doses substantially lower than those used in younger patients, and to monitor carefully for side-effects.

Thioridazine is commonly preferred to chlorpromazine in this age group because it is less sedating and there are fewer extra-pyramidal symptoms, but hypotension is more common. Given this man's eye problems, it is probably best to avoid chlorpromazine, however, because of its potential side-effects of pigmentary retinitis. Anxiolytic medications, such as benzodiazepines, should be used less liberally than in younger patients because of their propensity to cause delirium in elderly patients. Some paraphrenic patients are poorly compliant with medication, and remain floridly psychotic with adverse effects on their health and their family, and they may require treatment with depot medication.

5. Paraphrenia is a chronic condition requiring, in most cases, treatment for the rest of the patient's life. Drug treatment may be successful in reducing the florid manifestations of the initial episode, but in many cases it does not abolish delusional beliefs completely. However, patients seem to be able to co-exist with their delusions which are not obvious unless enquired into, and which do not interfere with day-to-day life. In general, those patients who present with a short history of florid illness which responds quickly to early treatment do better than those with a longer history, major sensory deficits, or evidence of cerebro-vascular disease. Non-compliance with medication is another important predictor of outcome.

Case 2

A 20-year-old woman who works as a graphic designer presents, and gives an 18-month history of 'panic attacks' of increasing severity and frequency, particularly over the last three months. During attacks, her stomach starts knotting up, she gets a queasy feeling in her throat and she feels nauseated, though she does not vomit. She also finds herself short of breath, with palpitations, hot flushes and sweaty palms and notices a haziness in front of her eyes. The attacks are usually of an hour or so in duration, and are now occurring daily. During attacks she feels that she will vomit in public, and therefore be embarrassed, but denies related fears that she might die, or suffer some other serious consequences. Attacks are particularly likely to happen when she is going out socially, or when she is travelling on public transport, and she now avoids these activities as far as possible. Her social life is consequently very limited, and she is finding it difficult to travel to and from work.

She remembers vividly an incident at the age of six years when she vomited in a large department store in the company of her mother and felt acutely embarrassed. She says her mother does not remember this incident. She has only vomited on a very few occasions since then, when physically unwell, and remembers being acutely distressed on each occasion.

Her father is a 45-year-old travel agent who is well, apart from glaucoma. Her mother is a 41-year-old physiotherapist who is well, but has had a recent hysterectomy. There is a younger brother aged 11 years who has recently been suffering from school refusal. She gets on well with her parents and there is no family history of psychiatric illness.

She was born and bred in London, with no obstetric or neonatal complications, and she describes a healthy, happy childhood, apart from some separation anxiety on first going to school. She enjoyed school and did relatively well, leaving at the age of 16 years to attend a further education college for a course in graphic design. On finishing the course, she took up work in central London, in a position she enjoys, but has found travelling to and from work increasingly distressing. She rarely uses alcohol, fearing that it will make her sick, and smokes very occasionally. She is heterosexual, and currently lives with her steady boyfriend. She describes her boyfriend as supportive and helpful through her current difficulties, although her problems are causing some strain between them. At interview she is brightly dressed, co-operative, and forthcoming with information. She does not appear unduly anxious during the interview, but does describe recent feelings of depression in response to the limitations imposed by her symptoms. There are no biological features of depression, and she denies any suicidal intent. There is no evidence of formal thought disorder, or abnormal experiences or beliefs. She did report an increasing tendency to believe that people are gossiping about her, over the last six months. She is cognitively intact.

She has attended the out-patient clinic hoping that you will be able to offer some psychological treatment, and has said that she will decline any drug treatment fearing that it will make her sick.

Questions

1. What is your diagnosis?
2. How do you relate the biological and psychological theories of aetiology for panic disorder?
3. How would you treat this patient?
4. What is the relationship between agoraphobia and panic disorder.
5. What other symptoms might a patient with panic disorder present to a psychiatrist?

Answers

1. In a 20-year-old woman with an 18-month history of intermittent attacks which involve autonomic symptoms, intense apprehension, and a fear of embarrassing herself through vomiting, and which have led to avoidance, the diagnosis is very probably panic disorder, in the DSM-III-R classification. ICD-9 does not distinguish between generalized anxiety and episodic anxiety as in panic attacks. It may be necessary to exclude organic diagnoses such as hyperthyroidism or phaeochromocytoma with appropriate examination and investigations. She displays some depressive features, and panic symptoms may arise as a result of a depressive illness, but the relative severity of the panic and depressive symptoms, and the chronology, all suggest that a primary depressive illness is unlikely in this patient.
2. Research has shown many biological differences between patients with panic disorder and controls. Some of this evidence is contradictory, and it is difficult to integrate it all into

a single biological model. Among the features demonstrated have been neurotransmitter abnormalities, abnormal responses to sodium lactate infusion, cardiac abnormalities, and evidence of increased sympathetic tone, such as a higher cardiac rate and increased beat-to-beat fluctuation. Respiratory abnormalities are also seen in patients with panic disorder, so that end tidal volume is commonly lowered either at rest or on exercise. However, it is difficult for any of the biological theories to explain the episodic nature of panic attacks. A psychological model has been proposed which suggests that patients with panic disorder are either more aware of bodily sensations or have relatively minor organic problems causing an excess of bodily sensations. The major difference between them and controls is their tendency to interpret these bodily sensations as evidence of threatening events, such as heart attacks. This generates anxiety, which in turn, through a variety of mechanisms (such as hyperventilation and chest muscle tension) produces further abnormal bodily sensations, and therefore sets up a vicious circle of positive feedback. This model both explains how a panic attack might arise, and also suggests that modification of the faulty cognitions which underlie the cycle may be an effective form of psychological treatment.

3. Panic disorder has been shown to respond to a number of different anxiolytic drugs, particularly alprazolam, and the MAOIs e.g. phenelzine. Although these can provide short-term symptomatic relief, they may simply serve to maintain the problem in the long-term. Whichever drug is used, relapse rates on discontinuing the drug are very high. For this reason attention has been directed towards psychological treatments which are claimed to offer long-term benefits.

This patient had already indicated that she would be very reluctant to consider drug treatment, and yet her symptoms appear increasingly disabling. Without treatment it is possible that they may lead to severely restrictive agoraphobia. She is therefore a good candidate for cognitive behavioural psychotherapy, which could either be offered by oneself, or for which she could be referred as appropriate. The principles underlying this treatment are that the fundamental misattributions of physical symptoms as evidence of illness should be identified and challenged by use of diaries, behavioural experiments, and homework assignments. There is good evidence for the effectiveness of this treatment.

4. In the DSM-III-R classification, panic disorder is classified as occurring with or without agoraphobia, and there is a separate category for agoraphobia without a history of panic disorder. For some patients with panic disorder, the attacks are limited to certain circumstances such as being alone outside the home, being in a crowded or enclosed space, or being on a high bridge. The fear of experiencing a panic attack may well lead to avoidance of these situations and consequently put severe restrictions on mobility; this amounts to agoraphobia secondary to panic disorder. Other patients do not experience panic in such particular circumstances, or, if they do, they do not avoid these situations to the same degree. A third group, those with agoraphobia without panic disorder, are severely restricted in their mobility outside the home, not because they fear panic attacks, which they do not have, but for some other reasons, such as a fear of loss of control over bladder or bowel function, or a fainting episode.

This patient displays symptoms of panic attacks with a degree of secondary agoraphobia. It would be important, during the course of any psychological treatment, to identify and challenge her avoidances, and to gradually expose her to hitherto avoided situations. Any course of treatment which does not deal with avoidance, whether overt or subtle, is unlikely to succeed in relieving the panic symptoms.

5. The DSM-III-R criteria for panic disorder lists 13 symptoms, of which a minimum of four are required during at least one attack. Ten of these 13 symptoms refer to bodily sensations, such as shortness of breath, sweating, nausea, or chest pain. In cases where the physical symptoms are emphasized, and the accompanying fear is either not fully recognized by the patient, or not elicited in the interview, the patient may well present to a medical out-patient clinic for investigation of episodic physical symptoms. Panic disorder can commonly be diagnosed amongst patients attending a cardiac clinic as

atypical chest pain, and, similarly, the episodic palpitations, shortness of breath or choking sensations may all lead to medical referrals. One of the important tasks of a liaison psychiatry service is to demonstrate to general physicians the frequency of panic disorder amongst their patients, and to provide effective treatment.

Case 3

A 39-year-old married woman who is currently an out-patient has just been seen. She reports having felt profoundly depressed each winter for the last ten years. She would begin to get depressed each October, and then her mood would get gradually lower until January, after which it slowly improved, resolving fully by March. During the winter, together with low moods, she would notice anhedonia, excessive sleep, a lack of energy, loss of interest, social withdrawal, decreased libido, carbohydrate craving, and substantial weight gain. She says that she has never had any depression during the summer months, and had never noticed any hypomanic swings. She had not noticed the seasonal pattern of her mood swings until two or three years previously when reading an article in a woman's magazine, which led her to seek treatment.

She is an only child. Her father was a civil servant, who died when she was 21 years old, and her mother is a housewife without medical problems, who is now 58 years old. A paternal uncle had required ECT for several depressive episodes, but there was no other family history of psychiatric illness.

She was born prematurely but suffered no lasting effects. Her childhood was healthy and happy, with many friends, both at home and at school. She was academically bright, gaining eight 'O' levels and three 'A' levels, but described her years in the sixth form college as difficult because of a poor relationship with her father. She went on to train as a teacher and has taught in a local secondary school since she qualified. She married a fellow teacher whom she met at college, and by whom she has twin boys, now aged 10 years, and both well. She smokes ten cigarettes a day, but does not drink.

She has had no serious medical illnesses, but on two occasions, two years apart, before she developed her winter depression, she said she was 'nearly anorexic' with substantial weight loss, excess dieting, and laxative abuse. She was not referred for psychiatric treatment at this time, being supported throughout by her general practitioner and a local self-help group, with some benefit.

She describes her personality as a perfectionist, who is irritable when she cannot get her own way. At interview, she is smartly dressed, and fully co-operative. Although superficially cheerful, she soon becomes tearful on recounting the experiences of the previous winters, and clearly describes how she feels she has missed out on life. Apart from this, there are no depressive features currently evident, it now being March. No abnormalities are evident in her speech, thought form, or perception, and her cognition is intact.

Questions

1. What do you think is the matter with her?
2. How would you treat her?
3. What is the significance of hypomanic mood swing following a depressive episode?

Answers

1. This woman has had recurrent episodes of depression, which occur exclusively in the winter months, and which have a number of atypical features, such as hypersomnia and weight gain. In the last 10 years it has been suggested that patients with this picture may have a particular sub-type of depression labelled 'seasonal affective disorder', and she appears to fit the criteria. The characteristic features are (for the northern hemisphere) a gradual lowering of mood from the autumn months, which becomes maximal in January or February, and which resolves with the coming of spring. There is often a mild hypomanic spell following the resolution of the depression, but this is rarely severe enough to

cause functional impairment, or to bring the patient into contact with psychiatric services at that time. As well as the low mood, the depression is characterized by such atypical features as hypersomnia, and weight gain secondary to carbohydrate craving. Although suicidal thoughts may occur, suicide attempts appear to be uncommon, at least in comparison with more typical episodes of depression. The validity of this diagnostic category has not yet been fully accepted, and many psychiatrists would simply classify this woman as somebody suffering with recurrent depression, with previous episodes of eating disorder.

2. Many patients with this seasonal pattern, together with mood swings, spend most of each winter on antidepressant medication with little obvious benefit. There is evidence that phototherapy with full spectrum lights offering a light intensity and pattern similar to that of natural sunlight, can bring about a rapid response in elevating mood. Patients are required to sit fairly close to a suitable light source for up to six hours a day, at times designed to extend the period of natural daylight. Improvement, if it is to occur, is usually evident within 5–7 days, and a return to lowered mood follows the withdrawal of light treatment by a similar period. Because this treatment, being more 'natural' than drug treatment, is attractive to patients, many patients with a disorder or recurrent depression may present claiming that it has an exclusively seasonal pattern. A detailed initial assessment will usually reveal that this is not the case, but a trial of light treatment may be required if the diagnosis remains in doubt. Lightboxes are available for purchase through a variety of companies, and do not require a prescription, but cost several hundred pounds each, a price beyond the range of many patients.

3. In patients with full-blown bipolar affective disorder, a typical manic episode may follow rapidly upon an episode of depression. Milder, and much shorter manic mood swings may occasionally be noticed in depressed patients following the resolution of the depression, whether this is spontaneous, or brought about by antidepressant treatment. In those patients where such changes are spontaneous, but do not amount to a full-blown manic episode, the label 'bipolar

II' affective disorder has been applied. Where the hypomanic mood swings follow treatment with antidepressants or ECT, this may constitute evidence for predisposition towards bipolar affective disorder, while not justifying the application of the diagnosis. In some patients, antidepressant treatment or ECT may actually precipitate a full-blown manic or hypomanic episode, which then requires treatment in its own right. In the case of seasonal affective disorder, a short lived and generally mild episode of activity and elevated mood is one of the typical features of the condition.

Case 4

A 29-year-old second generation immigrant of Nigerian extraction who is currently an in-patient detained under the Mental Health Act (MHA) has just been examined. He has had several previous admissions to hospital and since the last one he had been attending the occupational therapy department as a day-patient. Over the week preceding the current admission he had been noted by the occupational therapy staff to be increasingly noisy, disruptive, and sexually disinhibited. Despite an increase in the dose of his oral medication (trifluoperazine) the symptoms had worsened sufficiently for him to require admission under section. He says that he had been fully compliant with his medication, but he had noticed himself becoming increasingly 'high' following a period of friction between himself and his strict, disciplinarian father.

He is the fourth of eight siblings, two of whom have required out-patient treatment for depressive episodes. His parents are both well, his father working as a preacher in a local pentecostal church, and his mother as a housewife. He gets on well with his mother but finds the restrictions placed on his life by his father irksome. He has had no serious medical problem in the past, but has required admission to this psychiatric hospital on four previous occasions over the last seven years for similar symptoms. He had been treated with a variety of medications, details of which he is unable to recall, except that he does say 'I wasn't able to take lithium'. He has never had ECT. He was born in Coventry, his parents having arrived in Britain three years previously, and has moved several times with his family as his father took up different church positions. He tells you he enjoyed his childhood, but did not do well at school. He left school at 16 years of age to take up work as an office clerk, and continued in this post, although dissatisfied with the work, until his first psychiatric admission. He has not worked since, and between admissions lives at home with his parents on social security benefits. Previous attempts at rehabilitation and gradual re-introduction to work have all been curtailed by subsequent admissions. He describes his personality as a relaxed happy-go-lucky type, who can be the life-and-soul of the party when he is feeling good.

At interview, he is dressed in grubby, casual clothes, and he appears only mildly agitated and restless. However, while waiting to be interviewed in the company of nursing staff, and after interview, it was noticed that he had been declaiming loud monologues with a lot of motor agitation. One of the nurses accompanying him reported that he had woken all the patients on the ward last night by noisy bath-taking. Although he did not appear so at the time of interview, he described himself as 'high and elated'. He denied any depressive symptoms or suicidal ideas, and reported that he had been sleeping and eating normally. This was confirmed by the nursing staff. His speech appeared normal in rate, rhythm and intonation during the interview, but again, as soon as he was not being observed, he started talking loudly and rapidly on a variety of things including African nationalism and the Bible. He was pre-occupied with the fact that he was high again, but no formal thought disorder was evident. He did, however, report the experience of having his thoughts removed from his head and broadcast to other people around him. He also reported hearing infrequently the voice of a small girl calling his name and telling him to do things. He was cognitively intact. As to insight, he was aware that he was not his normal self, and agreed that he needed treatment and that being in hospital was the best place for him.

Questions

1. Summarize his presentation and give your differential diagnosis.
2. How would you treat him?
3. What is his prognosis?
4. If he agrees to remain on the ward, but refuses treatment, to what extent can he be compelled to accept it?
5. If this patient's urine drug screen unexpectedly shows that he had smoked cannabis, how would you see the relationship between his cannabis use and his illness?

Answers

1. This is a 29-year-old single man with recurrent episodes of psychotic illness, in which there is evidence of overactivity, agitation, restlessness, possible pressure of speech, flight of ideas, abnormalities of thought possession, and second person auditory hallucinations. There is a family history of affective disorder. The current admission appears to be precipitated by an exacerbation of the continuing friction between himself and his father.

   Assuming that organic causes have been excluded by physical examination and appropriate investigation, and drug-induced psychosis excluded by a drug history and urine drug screen, the differential diagnosis lies between schizophrenia, bipolar affective disorder, and schizoaffective disorder. He displays a number of features suggesting schizophrenia, particularly the first rank symptoms of thought withdrawal and thought broadcasting, and the apparent deterioration of personality requiring him to live at home and preventing him from working. There are also, however, some manic features in his agitation, disinhibition, and elated mood. However, the presence of first rank symptoms does not exclude the possibility of a manic episode. This almost equal mixture of features of schizophrenia and manic illness suggests that an intermediate diagnosis, namely schizoaffective disorder, may be the most appropriate. There is controversy about the validity of this diagnostic category, and uncertainty about the criteria by which it should be identified, and the term 'schizoaffective' has been used in a variety of different senses.

2. It would be important before prescribing medication for him to clarify what he has been taking before admission, and what he has been given on previous admissions which proved effective or ineffective, as the case may be. Whatever neuroleptic medication had seemed to benefit him most in the past should be chosen, and, given his current levels of agitation, it might be best to use one with more sedating properties, such as chlorpromazine. His claim that he had been compliant with medication should be checked by discussion with his parents, and with the staff who see him between admissions, and if there is doubt about his continued compliance, the use of a depot neuroleptic such as flupenthixol should be considered. Lithium may be of value in preventing relapses of schizoaffective disorder, though it appears to be less effective than in bipolar disorder. However, his statement that he could not take lithium is worrying, as it suggests that there was some contraindication that would need to be confirmed. If it was true that lithium was not suitable for him, then carbamazapine might be tried on an empirical basis, although its value in schizoaffective disorder has not been demonstrated. It is important that his drug treatment is accompanied by a carefully structured programme of rehabilitation. He has now been unemployed for many years, and unless he can be reintegrated into the working world soon, he is likely to remain unemployed for the rest of his life. A rehabilitation plan involving the disablement resettlement officer of the local job centre, and the occupational therapy department, therefore needs to be part of his current treatment. In addition, since friction with his father may be a fact of precipitating relapses, work with his family to reduce the levels of Expressed Emotion at home, and possibly consider his moving out of home to live in a hostel or other accommodation, should be undertaken.

3. In general, the prognosis of schizoaffective disorder is said to be intermediate between that of bipolar affective disorder and schizophrenia. However, the fact that this man has already had several admissions before the age of 30 years,

and that between admissions he does not appear to function well, and that his relapses seem to be easily precipitated by social stresses, all indicate a poor prognosis. This is also suggested by the failure of previous attempts at rehabilitation.

4. In England and Wales, under the Mental Health Act 1983, both Section 2 and Section 3 empower a responsible medical officer to authorize drug treatment against the patient's will. Since Section 2 is a short-term section intended for assessment, it is preferable, but not required, that patients be transferred to a Section 3 before such treatment is given. Section 3 allows for the administration of drug treatment for a period of three months in the first instance. If, after that time, the patient still does not consent, Section 58 requires that a second medical opinion be obtained through the Mental Health Act Commission, to approve a plan of continued treatment.

   This second opinion requirement also applies to ECT, if it is refused, from the beginning of the treatment course. If it is judged that ECT is needed on an emergency basis, in depressive stupor for example, Section 62 (also see p.118) empowers the responsible medical officer to give one or two applications of treatment while arranging a second opinion. Other, infrequently used treatments (currently psychosurgery and hormonal treatment to alter sex drive) require, under Section 57, *both* consent and a second opinion.

   If emergency treatment is required to prevent serious risk to himself or to others, this would also be justifiable under common law, but it would be important to set in motion the relevant provisions of the MHA legislation at the same time.

5. The relationship between cannabis use and psychosis is a controversial one. There is little doubt that cannabis can induce an acute intoxication, with euphoria and hallucinations, particularly in the visual modality. This usually clears after a few days of abstinence, but some patients with a urine drug screen positive for cannabis remain psychotic for much longer than this. It has been suggested that there is a characteristic 'cannabis psychosis', but the evidence does

not support the concept of a specific set of symptoms defining a psychosis associated with cannabis use. There is evidence from a large Scandinavian follow-up study that heavy cannabis use may increase the risk of developing schizophrenia, and it seems that in patients with established psychotic illnesses (as here) cannabis may precipitate relapses. Such patients (and their families) should be strongly advised to avoid the use of cannabis and other drugs. Finally, the association may, of course, be spurious. In some inner city areas, cannabis use is very widespread, and a high proportion of a random sample of general hospital attenders will show evidence of cannabis intake. It is quite possible that in this patient his cannabis use and psychosis are unconnected, or even that he took the cannabis in response to his psychotic symptoms, in an attempt to calm himself down.

Case 5

A 45-year-old woman who is currently an in-patient, detained under the Mental Health Act has just been seen. She has had a great many previous psychiatric admissions, and since the last one ended 10 months ago, she had been well, on phenelzine, and attending out-patients regularly. She says that on the day before admission, she had experienced a sudden onset of 'black despair' and a profound sense of hopelessness, accompanied by suicidal urges. She visited her general practitioner but ran off in tears half-way through the consultation. Her general practitioner was sufficiently concerned to summon the police, who found her in the local market place, cutting at her forearm with a piece of glass. They took her under Section 136 to the police station, where she was seen by a psychiatrist who arranged her admission.

She says that since admission her mood has very rapidly returned to normal, and she now feels entirely well. When she is asked about events preceding this episode, it emerges that the doctor she usually saw in outpatients was about to move to another post, and she complains bitterly that 'They keep doing this to me: things go well and then they move on'.

She is one of a pair of non-identical twins and three other children, born to a local farmer and his wife. Her twin had an episode of depression 10 years ago but is now well, and there is no other family psychiatric history.

She says she never got on with her parents, particularly her father, who was rigid, authoritarian, cold and demanding. As a consequence, her childhood was very unhappy, and made worse by an episode of sexual abuse she suffered at the hands of an uncle when aged 12 years. She did poorly at school, where her headmaster had been sufficiently concerned about her to want her to see a child psychiatrist, but her parents refused. On leaving school, she took up work as a nursing assistant, but soon afterwards suffered the first of many psychiatric admissions, and she has not worked since. With her repeated admissions, she gradually became estranged from her parents, and 10 years ago moved in with an elderly man she met as a fellow-patient on the ward. He has proved supportive and concerned.

Her many admissions have all been relatively short, with a presentation similar to the current one, and she has been treated with a wide range of different drugs. On one occasion, five years ago, she was admitted for a longer period and underwent a course of ECT. Many admissions have been under Section.

At interview, she is casually dressed and co-operative, with an immature child-like manner. There is no abnormality of movement, but it can be seen that her sleeveless dress exposes multiple old scars on both forearms, and more recent cigarette burns on the back of her left hand. She notices that these are obvious and admits, with a smile, that she did it herself 'so I could feel better'. There is no current evidence of depressed mood, and she reports sleeping and eating well. No psychotic phenomena are evident, and she is cognitively intact. She says that she is not ill, she just over-reacts, and that now she wants to go home.

Questions

1. What diagnosis would you consider?

2. How do you define an abnormal personality?
3. What aetiological factors are relevant in the development of personality disorder?
4. How would you manage this patient?

Answers

1. The absence of current psychopathology, the recent history of abrupt onset and rapid resolution of dramatic symptoms, and the long-term history of similar frequent brief admissions, beginning in adolescence, all suggest that this patient has a personality disorder rather than a current Axis I illness. She may have had a superimposed depressive episode in the past, and she has a family history of affective illness, so care needs to be taken to exclude a current depressive episode as well as a personality disorder, but the lack of symptoms on mental state examination indicate this is unlikely.

   In the ICD-9 classification, the most appropriate category would be hysterical personality disorder, given her apparent dependence on others, and the theatrical nature of some of her behaviours. A history of sexual frigidity would provide confirmatory evidence. The DSM-III-R equivalent would be histrionic personality disorder, or perhaps, given her self-mutilatory behaviour, affective instability and response to perceived rejection, borderline personality disorder.

2. Although individuals' personalities vary widely, the definition of what separates normal and abnormal personalities is far from clear. In a dimensional approach, the differences are seen as quantitative—an abnormal personality simply has an excess of one or more normal personality traits. However, both DSM-III-R and ICD-9 use a categorical approach, suggesting that there are qualitative differences. The essence of the difference is that those with personality disorder display deeply ingrained maladaptive patterns of behaviour which are recognizable by adolescence and continue through much of adult life. This behaviour leads either the patient or others to suffer adverse consequences.

3. Psychodynamic theories intended to explain the development of normal personality can be applied to provide hypotheses for the ways in which personality disorders arise. The hypotheses are usually framed in terms of the effect of disruptive experiences during early childhood development, which either arrests in a particular state, or renders the individual liable to regression to an immature stage of development when under stress. It is difficult, however, to find evidence to confirm or refute these hypotheses, and there is little to support the suggestion that specific types of disturbance in childhood lead to various different personality disorders.

Other explanations emphasize the effects of early environment, but in different ways. The behaviourists explain personality as a set of behavioural traits developed and maintained by environmental conditioning, while social learning theorists emphasize the role of social reinforcement and cultural expectations.

An alternative type of explanation altogether emphasizes the genetic contribution to personality, but there is scanty evidence for or against, except in the case of antisocial personality disorder. Even here, uncertainty about diagnostic criteria has led to a mass of contradictory evidence, though twin and adoption studies do suggest some genetic contribution.

A further type of explanation emphasizes organic aspects, suggesting that either minimal brain damage or delay in cerebral maturation might underlie the behavioural features of personality disorder. This may be true to an extent for antisocial personality, but there is little evidence to support it as an explanation of all personality abnormalities.

4. Although hospital admissions may be necessary in a crisis, as in this case, it is best avoided where possible, as it may prove counterproductive in the long-term. Drugs are unlikely to be helpful unless there is a superimposed Axis I disorder, and there is a risk of inducing dependence and abuse. They may, however, have a role in the short-term management of acute stress. Psychological approaches are therefore the treatment of choice. Individual or group

psychodynamic psychotherapy has a place for some personality disorders, but is both difficult and unsuccessful in antisocial personality, for which therapeutic communities are preferable. When used, it is likely to be needed over a longer period than that customary in treating neurosis, and the aim may need to be more limited. Some patients cannot tolerate the demands of psychoanalytic psychotherapy, and a long-term supportive approach may be more suitable. In this patient's case, her reaction to the departure of her doctor indicates she should be seen over the long term, though not necessarily very frequently, by a therapist who is less likely to move away.

Index

Note: In keeping with the format of the book, the majority of references are to the complete case.